BINGE-EATING DISORDER

Binge-Eating Disorder

Clinical Foundations and Treatment

James E. Mitchell
Michael J. Devlin
Martina de Zwaan
Scott J. Crow
Carol B. Peterson

THE GUILFORD PRESS
New York   London

To Albert J. Stunkard, MD
and
Robert L. Spitzer, MD

Library of Congress Cataloging-in-Publication Data

Binge-eating disorder : clinical foundations and treatment / James E. Mitchell . . . [et al.].
       p. ; cm.
    Includes bibliographical references and index.
    ISBN-13: 978-1-59385-594-9 (pbk. : alk. paper)
    ISBN-10: 1-59385-594-X (pbk. : alk. paper)
    1. Compulsive eating. 2. Compulsive eating—Treatment. 3. Cognitive therapy. I. Mitchell, James E. (James Edward), 1947–
    [DNLM: 1. Bulimia. 2. Bulimia—therapy. 3. Cognitive Therapy. WM 175 B6128 2008]
    RC552.C65B53 2008
    616.85′26—dc22
                                                            2007018388

About the Authors

James E. Mitchell, MD, is NRI/Lee A. Christofferson MD Professor and Chair of the Department of Clinical Neuroscience at the University of North Dakota School of Medicine and Health Sciences and President of the Neuropsychiatric Research Institute. Dr. Mitchell focuses primarily on research in the areas of eating disorders and obesity. He is past president of the Academy for Eating Disorders and the Eating Disorders Research Society and is on the editorial board of the *International Journal of Eating Disorders*. Dr. Mitchell has published more than 300 scientific articles and has either authored or edited 12 books.

Michael J. Devlin, MD, is Associate Professor of Clinical Psychiatry at Columbia University College of Physicians and Surgeons and Associate Director of the Eating Disorders Research Unit at the New York State Psychiatric Institute. His major academic interest is in the diagnosis and treatment of patients with eating disorders. Dr. Devlin is an active member of the Academy for Eating Disorders and is past president of that organization. He serves on the editorial boards of two journals, the *International Journal of Eating Disorders* and *Eating Behaviors*. In addition to research in eating disorders, Dr. Devlin is active in medical student education and in the training and supervision of psychiatry residents, particularly in cognitive-behavioral therapy.

Martina de Zwaan, MD, is Professor and Head of the Department of Psychosomatic Medicine and Psychotherapy at the University Hospital of Erlangen, Germany. She is the author of numerous scientific and clinical papers on the subject of eating disorders, mainly bulimia nervosa, binge-eating disorder, and obesity.

Scott J. Crow, MD, is Professor of Psychiatry at the University of Minnesota. His research examines the course, outcome, and treatment of eating disorders and obesity. Dr. Crow is the recipient of an Independent Scientist Award (from the National Institute of Mental Health) focusing on the course, outcome, and treatment of eating disorders. He is past president of the Academy for Eating Disorders and director of the Eating Disorder/Assessment Core of the Minnesota Obesity Center.

Carol B. Peterson, PhD, is Research Associate/Assistant Professor in the Eating Disorders Research Program at the University of Minnesota, where her investigations have focused on the assessment, diagnosis, and treatment of bulimia nervosa, anorexia nervosa, binge-eating disorder, and obesity. She has authored over 50 articles and book chapters and has served as an investigator on several federally funded grants. Dr. Peterson is also Adjunct Assistant Professor in the Department of Psychology at the University of Minnesota and has a part-time private practice in which she specializes in the treatment of eating disorders.

Preface

The fourth edition of the *Diagnostic and Statistical Manual of Mental Disorders* (DSM-IV; American Psychiatric Association, 1994) contained an Appendix B entitled "Criteria Sets and Axes Provided for Further Study." One such criteria set was for binge-eating disorder (BED). It was not clear what impact the inclusion of the BED criteria in DSM-IV would have on the field. However, soon a number of research groups became very interested in this problem, and as you will see in the pages ahead, they have committed significant amounts of research time to further understanding this condition. A fairly extensive literature has thus accumulated. It ranges from basic studies looking at psychobiological changes, through epidemiological studies of prevalence in clinical and community samples, and treatment studies focusing on both pharmacotherapy and psychotherapy approaches. The five of us who authored this text have been among this group of investigators and have contributed to this literature.

The purpose of this book is twofold: first, to provide useful clinical information for practicing clinicians about the diagnosis and treatment of this condition, along with a manual for an evidence-based treatment; and second, to review the literature that has developed on this condition over the last dozen or so years, suggesting possible future avenues for research. Part II of this book comprises a cognitive-behavioral treatment manual for BED. Cognitive-behavioral therapy has been used in various forms at various centers, and appears to represent the best available treatment that we have for BED. This particular manual was developed at the University of Minnesota and updated more recently by investigators at both the University of Minnesota and the Neuropsychiatric Research Institute in Fargo, North Dakota. As will be described in the Introduction to This Treatment Program in Part II, the manual has now been used in clinical practice for the last 10 years as well as in two randomized treatment trials (Peterson et al., 1998, 2001, 2006).

In thinking back about those individuals most involved in the development of the criteria for BED, two in particular come to mind and we wish to acknowledge them. The first is Albert J. (Mickey) Stunkard, MD, a Professor of Psychiatry at the University of Pennsylvania. Mickey has contributed much to the study of obesity over the years. He described BED in 1959, although the problem was largely neglected for decades afterward. The second is Robert L. Spitzer, MD, a Professor at the New York State Psychiatric Institute and Columbia University. Bob had been the primary architect of the DSM-III and the DSM-III-R, and regularly met with the eating disorders committee charged with examining the diagnostic criteria for DSM-IV. That group met at Columbia on a regular basis over several years. Over that period of time, Bob advocated for creating a new disorder. He originally termed it "compulsive overeating," and when he first introduced the idea, most members of the committee were skeptical about the development of such a criteria set for the DSM system. However, Bob persevered, and over the period of years that the group met, he oversaw the development of a reasonably large body of data supporting the construct of BED. By the time that group had finished its work, most members of the committee were convinced that indeed BED was likely an important disorder.

We offer the current text as a clinical guide and a briefing on the state of the art and science in this field. We hope clinicians will find this material clinically informative and the manual useful in their practices. We hope researchers will also find this literature review helpful and the tentative suggestions for further research provocative.

JAMES E. MITCHELL, MD
MICHAEL J. DEVLIN, MD
MARTINA DE ZWAAN, MD
SCOTT J. CROW, MD
CAROL B. PETERSON, PhD

References

American Psychiatric Association. (1994). *Diagnostic and statistical manual of mental disorders* (4th ed.). Washington, DC: Author.

Peterson, C. B., Mitchell, J. E., Crow, S. J., Crosby, R. D., & Wonderlich, S. A. (2006, August). *A randomized comparison trial of group treatment models for binge eating disorder*. Paper presented at the annual meeting of the Eating Disorders Research Society, Port Douglas, Queensland, Australia.

Peterson, C. B., Mitchell, J. E., Engbloom, S., Nugent, S., Mussell M. P., Crow, S. J., et al. (2001). Self-help versus therapist-led group cognitive-behavioral treatment of binge eating disorder at follow-up. *International Journal of Eating Disorders, 30*(4), 363–374.

Peterson, C. B., Mitchell, J. E., Engbloom, S., Nugent, S., Mussell, M. P., & Miller, J. P. (1998). Group cognitive behavioral treatment of binge eating disorder: A comparison of therapist-led vs. self-help formats. *International Journal of Eating Disorders, 24*, 125–136.

Contents

I. WHAT WE KNOW ABOUT BINGE-EATING DISORDER AND ITS TREATMENT

1. Diagnosis and Epidemiology of Binge-Eating Disorder   3

2. Clinical Features, Longitudinal Course, and Psychopathology of Binge-Eating Disorder   13

3. Binge-Eating Disorder and Obesity   23

4. Eating Behavior, Psychobiology, Medical Risks, and Pharmacotherapy of Binge-Eating Disorder   35

5. Binge-Eating Disorder and Bariatric Surgery   49

6. Psychotherapy for Binge-Eating Disorder   58

7. Binge-Eating Disorder and the Future   70

II. A COGNITIVE-BEHAVIORAL TREATMENT PROGRAM FOR BINGE-EATING DISORDER

Introduction to This Treatment Program   75

Session-by-Session Therapist Guidelines   83

Patient Materials: Session-by-Session Handouts and Worksheets   109

References   189

Index   209

PART I

What We Know about Binge-Eating Disorder and Its Treatment

CHAPTER 1

Diagnosis and Epidemiology
of Binge-Eating Disorder

In 1959 Stunkard published the clinical observation that some obese individuals report having distressing episodes of overeating that they experience as outside of their control. Stunkard characterized an eating binge as "having an orgiastic quality" and noted that "enormous amounts of food are consumed in relatively short periods." He noticed that the eating binge is "frequently related to a specific precipitating event, and is regularly followed by severe discomfort and self-condemnation." Forty years later Stunkard's clinical observation led to the delineation of binge-eating disorder (BED).

BED has been included in the appendix of the fourth edition of the *Diagnostic and Statistical Manual of Mental Disorders* (DSM-IV; American Psychiatric Association, 1994) as a disorder for further study and is also included as an example of an eating disorder not otherwise specified (EDNOS). The introduction of BED to DSM-IV has stimulated much research over the past decade as well as many critical questions concerning the utility of this new diagnosis. There is no respective diagnostic category in the 10th revision of the *International Classification of Diseases* (ICD-10; World Health Organization, 1992).

The diagnostic criteria currently recommended for BED are presented in Table 1.1. In the current DSM-IV criteria, no distinction is made between obese and nonobese binge eaters. It is important to keep in mind that in clinical settings, the majority of persons with BED have varying degrees of obesity, even though the diagnosis is not limited to overweight or obese individuals (Spitzer et al., 1993a; see Chapter 3 for additional discussion).

Diagnostic Criteria

The definition of a binge-eating episode in DSM-IV is identical for both bulimia nervosa (BN) and BED, including the requirements of the ingestion of an unusually large amount of food

TABLE 1.1. Proposed Diagnostic Criteria for BED

A. Recurrent episodes of binge eating. An episode of binge eating is characterized by both of the following:

    (1) eating, in a discrete period of time (e.g., within any 2-hour period), an amount of food that is definitely larger than most people would eat during a similar period of time under similar circumstances

    (2) a sense of lack of control during the episodes (e.g., a feeling that one cannot stop eating or control what or how much one is eating)

B. The binge-eating episodes are associated with three (or more) of the following:

    (1) eating much more rapidly than normal

    (2) eating until feeling uncomfortably full

    (3) eating large amounts of food when not feeling physically hungry

    (4) eating alone because of being embarrassed by how much one is eating

    (5) feeling disgusted with oneself, depressed, or very guilty after overeating

C. Marked distress regarding binge eating is present.

D. The binge eating occurs, on average, at least 2 days a week for 6 months.

E. The binge eating is not associated with the regular use of inappropriate compensatory behaviors (e.g., purging, fasting, excessive exercise) and does not occur exclusively during the course of Anorexia Nervosa or Bulimia Nervosa.

Note. From American Psychiatric Association (2000). Copyright 2000 by the American Psychiatric Association. Reprinted by permission.

and a feeling of loss of control over the eating episode. The diagnosis is restricted to patients who have "objective" binge-eating episodes that are defined in quantitative rather than qualitative terms. How to properly assess binge eating remains particularly problematic. The Eating Disorder Examination (EDE—Cooper & Fairburn, 1987; Fairburn & Cooper, 1993), a semistructured interview developed to assess eating pathology, differentiates between subjective and objective binge-eating episodes, viewing the phenomenon from both the subject's (subjective) and the clinician's (objective) perspectives. In both types of binge eating a feeling of loss of control is required; in an objective episode the interviewer agrees with the patient that the amount of food is more than most people would eat under similar circumstances. The EDE also included the term "picking" or "nibbling," defined as eating in an unplanned and repetitive way between meals and snacks, without a sense of loss of control.

The Structured Inventory for Anorexic and Bulimic Eating Disorders (SIAB-EX—Fichter et al., 1998; Fichter & Quadflieg, 2001) can be used to assess binge-eating behavior in a structured way. This instrument differentiates between three types of binge eating: objective binge eating, subjective binge eating, and "atypical binge eating," also labeled as "grazing" or "constant overeating." The main characteristic of atypical binges is that food is not consumed in a short period of time but rather ingested, more or less continuously, throughout the day or during part of the day (e.g., in the evening). The amounts of food consumed are small, so that the activity does not constitute an eating binge in the strict sense of the word, and there is only a slight loss of control. The definition of atypical binge eating is unique to the SIAB-EX and is not covered by other published assessment instruments. Fichter and Quadflieg (2001) describe it as an "experimental scale" and consider their definitions of binge eating to be closer to the

DSM-IV criteria, which define binge eating as lasting for "a discrete period of time (e.g., within any 2-hour period)." In line with this definition, Marcus and colleagues (1992) reported that almost 25% of binge-eating episodes by obese binge eaters lasted an entire day, suggesting a great deal of variability. All-day binges appear to violate the DSM-IV specification of occurring "in a discrete period of time." Cooper and Fairburn (2003) acknowledge that it is particularly difficult to distinguish episodes of binge eating from "unstructured overeating." It is also sometimes difficult to determine whether the amounts eaten are truly large, and individuals are often unclear whether they experienced a sense of loss of control. For objective and especially subjective binge-eating episodes, the level of agreement is usually relatively low between self-report and interview assessment in individuals with BED. Interestingly, the self-report questionnaires produce lower frequencies of objective binge-eating episodes and subjective binge-eating episodes than the interview, which contrast with the results seen in BN (see de Zwaan et al., 2004). Nonetheless, the interviewer must be aware of these problems and make a judgment on the basis of the best available guidelines (Table 1.2).

TABLE 1.2. Definitions of Different Aspects of Eating Episodes

Term	Definition
Objective binge-eating episodes[a]	Eating an objectively large amount of food with a sense of loss of control (DSM-IV, EDE, SIAB).
Subjective binge-eating episodes	Eating a subjectively large amount of food with a sense of loss of control (EDE, SIAB).
Loss of control	Feeling that one cannot stop eating or control what or how much one is eating (DSM-IV, SIAB). Feeling driven or compelled to eat, unable to stop eating, unable to prevent the eating episode, no longer trying to control eating. Does not require the agreement of the subject (EDE).
Objectively large amount	More than the usual amount eaten under the circumstances (DSM-IV). Does not require the agreement of the subject (EDE).
Atypical eating binges	Eating more or less continuously throughout the day or during part of the day (e.g., in the evening). The amounts of food consumed are small, so that the activity does not constitute an eating binge in the strict sense of the word. There is only a slight loss of control (SIAB).
Duration of binge-eating episodes	Eating, in a discrete period of time (e.g., within any 2-hour period) (DSM-IV). An hour or more when the subject was not eating terminates a binge eating episode (EDE).
Picking, nibbling	Eating in an unplanned and repetitious way between meals and snacks without a sense of loss of control (EDE).
Snack	Episode of eating in which the amount eaten is modest, known at the outset with some certainty and without the repetitious element (EDE).

Note: DSM-IV, *Diagnostic and Statistical Manual of Mental Disorders* (4th ed.); EDE, Eating Disorder Examination; SIAB, Structured Inventory for Anorexic and Bulimic Eating Disorders.
[a]Required in DSM-IV for a diagnosis of BED.

Even though the concept of BED has strong face validity, content and construct validity are less well established especially concerning the usefulness of binge eating as the main symptom of BED. Distinguishing BED from other types of overeating is not straightforward, and in clinical practice many cases are difficult to classify. The diagnostic criteria for BED focus on days per week with binge-eating episodes rather than individual episodes, the rationale being that subjects with BED may have more difficulty recalling discrete binge-eating episodes than those with BN. In purging BN, binge-eating episodes can be defined by the presence of vomiting or laxative abuse that usually terminates the binge-eating episode, whereas with BED, the termination of the eating binge is not punctuated by such discrete, easily recalled behavior. Many patients, therefore, experience difficulties in precisely recalling and labeling discrete binge-eating episodes (Rossiter et al., 1992). Recent studies show that subjects without BED also recorded binge-eating episodes during a period of self-monitoring of food intake (Greeno et al., 2000; le Grange et al., 2001; Yanovski & Sebring, 1994). In addition, the binge-eating episodes of overweight individuals are generally not as large, and may differ in other important ways, from the binge eating described by patients with BN (Brody et al., 1994). Thus the single definition of a binge-eating episode for both disorders, as currently used in DSM-IV, may not fit clinical reality (Gladis et al., 1998b).

The extent to which DSM-IV criteria make meaningful distinctions between full and subthreshold eating disorders has been questioned, and it has been suggested that the diagnostic criteria should be broadened. Individuals with binge-eating problems often do not meet the frequency criterion of two binge days per week. There is evidence that subthreshold BED subjects do not differ significantly from subjects meeting full criteria. They frequently evidence the same risk for psychiatric distress, low self-esteem, impaired social adjustment, and overconcern with shape and weight (Crow et al., 2002; Striegel-Moore et al., 1998, 2000a; Wilson et al., 1993). This finding raises questions about the utility of the frequency requirement, which was arbitrarily chosen to match the BN frequency criterion. In addition, it has been suggested that individuals with BED who interpret the consumption of an objectively small amount of food as a "binge" could be considered more disturbed psychologically than those who use the term only for true "gorging" episodes (Beumont et al., 1994). Overall, there is no sharp demarcation between the full syndrome and the subthreshold groups, and consequently some recent treatment studies have included subthreshold cases.

Distress regarding binge eating is required for the diagnosis of BED. This "distress" includes unpleasant feelings during and after the binge-eating episode, as well as concerns about the long-term effect of the recurrent episodes on body weight and shape and self-esteem. The inclusion of this item in the diagnostic criteria was meant to minimize false positives. In Spitzer and colleagues' (1992) multisite field trial, removal of this item would have markedly increased the number of subjects meeting criteria for BED (by 10%, from 30.1 to 33.8%, in a weight control sample, and by more than 50%, from 2 to 4.6%, in a community sample). However, it is not entirely clear how to measure "marked distress"—a problem shared by the use of this criterion in many disorders in DSM-IV. Does it only require the patient's self-report about her or his emotional state, or does it require some impairment of the patient's functioning in social situations or at work due to binge eating? Also, it seems possible that this criterion identifies individuals with high levels of distress, in general. On the other hand, there are patients who meet all the other criteria for BED but simply deny distress.

Another area of concern is the risk of definitional overlap across related categories. The most problematic boundary is the one between BED and nonpurging BN. In both diagnostic categories there are recurrent binge-eating episodes in the absence of regular vomiting, laxative, or diuretic misuse. Nonpurging BN is diagnosed by the use of nonpurging compensatory behaviors such as "fasting," defined as not eating anything for 24 hours (which replaced the term "strict dieting" used in DSM-III-R; Spitzer et al., 1993a) or excessive exercising, which is difficult to define. Hay and Fairburn (1998) compared individuals with purging BN, nonpurging BN, and BED cross-sectionally and over the course of 1 year. They could not differentiate nonpurging BN and BED on present state features such as binge-eating frequency or eating-related and general psychopathology, but individuals with purging type BN had the most severe symptoms. Those with BED showed less temporal stability compared to those with nonpurging BN, and they had a more benign 1-year outcome. Purging and nonpurging BN were similar in temporal stability. The authors concluded that this difference in predictive validity justified the diagnostic distinction between nonpurging BN and BED. In addition, they suggested that bulimic eating disorders might exist on a continuum of clinical severity, from BN purging type (most severe), through BN nonpurging type (intermediate severity), to BED (least severe).

Psychosocial Risk Factors

Only retrospective risk studies of BED, conducted in community samples, are available. Fairburn and colleagues (1998) compared putative risk factors preceding the onset of BED in 52 women with BED, 104 without an eating disorder, 102 with BN, and 102 with other psychiatric disorders. Compared to women without eating disorders or other psychiatric disorders, women with BED revealed greater exposure to certain adverse childhood experiences, such as sexual or physical abuse and bullying and family problems (e.g., parental psychiatric disorder, parental criticism, lack of affection, underinvolvement, overprotection). Also, negative self-evaluation and shyness appear to increase the risk for BED, and exposure to risk factors for obesity (e.g., childhood obesity, critical comments by family about shape, weight, or eating) appears to be associated with BED. However, compared with BN, the risk factors for BED are weaker. Even vulnerability to obesity seems to be more pronounced in BN.

Striegel-Moore and colleagues (2002) reported that a history of sexual abuse was associated with BED in a community sample of black and white women obtained from the New England Women's Health Project. Interestingly, a history of sexual abuse was significantly more common in black women (66%) compared to white women (23.8%) with BED.

Alternative Diagnostic Classifications

The DSM-IV as well as the ICD-10 use categorical approaches to describe psychopathology, and the diagnostic criteria were derived through expert consensus. Revisions of these classification systems have changed the diagnostic criteria for eating disorders several times over the past 20 years. Given the continued debate about the diagnostic validity of BED (Cooper & Fairburn, 2003; Devlin et al., 2003; Wilfley et al., 2003; Wonderlich et al., 2003), researchers have tried to assess the optimal set of diagnostic criteria for it and to further examine its predictive and construct validity. Several studies have attempted to regroup the individual symptoms of eating disorders using sophisticated statistical models and have found subgroups of eating disorders with different symptom profiles that usually resemble the current classifications (Bulik et al., 2000; Hay et al., 1996; Keel et al., 2004; Stice & Agras, 1999; Williamson et al., 2002). However, dimensional models of eating disorders have been proposed (Hay & Fairburn, 1998; Stice & Agras, 1999; Tylka & Subich, 1999). Thus far, neither categorical nor dimensional models of eating disorders have been shown to adequately represent the full spectrum of disturbed eating behaviors (Williamson et al., 2005).

New statistical approaches also have been used, such as taxometric analyses, to determine if a diagnostic entity is best represented as a discrete category or dimensional construct occurring on a continuum with normal behavior. A recent taxometric analysis by Williamson and colleagues (2002) provided evidence that BED is qualitatively distinct from both normal-weight comparison subjects and obese non-binge-eating subjects. A second taxometric study by Joiner and colleagues also provided support for the distinction of BED (Joiner, 1999). In a recent review of diagnostic studies on eating disorders, Williamson and colleagues (2005) endorsed the validity of BED based on the limited but consistent finding of BED as a true taxonic entity.

Dysfunctional attitudes regarding eating, weight, and shape have consistently been shown to be significantly more pronounced in individuals with BED, compared to obese non-binge-eating individuals, and to show comparable values to individuals with BN. Masheb and Grilo (2000a) therefore have suggested incorporating these cognitive diagnostic criteria into the set of diagnostic criteria for BED.

Several authors have attempted to identify meaningful subtypes of BED (Grilo et al., 2001; Peterson et al., 1998a, 2005; Stice et al., 2001). These include subtypes by mood and substance use disorders, subtypes of dietary restraint versus dietary restraint combined with negative affect, and subtypes with and without a history of purging behavior. For example, Stice and colleagues (2001) reported that a subtype of BED characterized by high negative affect was marked by significantly greater concerns regarding weight and shape as well as significantly higher levels of associated psychiatric disturbance and social maladjustment. In addition, the high-negative-affect subgroup did not respond as well to treatment. Likewise, Peterson and colleagues (2005) reported that individuals with BED and a history of affective or substance use disorder may have a more severe form of the disorder. Similar results were observed by Grilo and colleagues (2001). Subtypes concerning the temporal sequence of onset of binge eating versus dieting are described in the next chapter.

A major criticism of BED as a clinically significant disorder has been the lack of treatment specificity. BED seems to respond to a variety of procedurally and conceptually different treatments, including weight loss treatment, which appears to be equally effective in reducing binge eating (Wilfley et al., 2003). Moreover, the phenomenon of binge eating has been reported to be unstable over time (Fairburn et al., 2000). Therefore, Stunkard and Allison (2003) have argued that the construct BED should be viewed as a marker of psychopathology in obese individuals rather than a distinct disorder.

In an interview study with 888 first-degree relatives of overweight and obese individuals with and without BED, Hudson and colleagues (2006) demonstrated that BED aggregates in families independently of obesity. A lifetime diagnosis of BED was found in 20.2% of the relatives of probands with BED and 9.6% of the relatives of probands without BED. This finding suggests that BED is caused, in part, by familial factors distinct from any additional familial factors for obesity. The result of this study somewhat contradicts the view of Stunkard and

Allison (2003) and supports the assumption that BED represents an etiologically distinct behavioral phenotype of obesity and not just a nonspecific eating pattern seen in some obese individuals.

Devlin and colleagues (2003) proposed various models to conceptualize binge eating and discussed the pros and cons of BED as a distinct eating disorder, as a variant of BN, as a behavioral subtype of obesity, and finally as an associated feature that emerges when two primary disorders (e.g., obesity and depression) coexist. The authors concluded that none of the models can be ruled out entirely.

In summary, studies have explored alternative diagnostic items, syndromal threshold, and durations of BED. Other studies have attempted to create meaningful clinical subtypes of BED, and some have questioned the current diagnostic classification systems and suggested new categorical and dimensional classification systems of eating disorders.

Epidemiology

A few prevalence studies have relied on two-stage interview methods, and there are no studies examining the incidence—that is, new cases per year—of BED in representative community samples (Striegel-Moore & Franko, 2003). BED appears to be quite common among subjects attending hospital-affiliated weight loss programs, including weight loss surgery, with an overall frequency of DSM-IV criteria of approximately 30% (de Zwaan et al., 2003b; Grissett & Fitzgibbon, 1996; Kuehnel & Wadden, 1994; Spitzer et al., 1992, 1993b; Yanovski et al., 1994), ranging from 7.5 to 47.4% (Ho et al., 1995). However, estimates based on interviews rather than self-reports are considerably lower, varying between 9% (Stunkard et al., 1996b) and 19% (Brody et al., 1994). BED is more common than BN and anorexia nervosa (AN) in the general population, with approximately a 2% prevalence (Basdevant et al., 1995; Cortufo et al., 1997; Favaro et al., 2003; French et al., 1999; Hay, 1998; Kinzl et al., 1999; Smith et al., 1998; Spitzer et al., 1992, 1993b; Striegel-Moore et al., 2003; Wade et al., 2006; Westenhöfer, 2001). In Spitzer and colleagues' (1992) first multisite study, interestingly, only half of the community sample with BED was obese (BMI > 27.5 kg/m^2); however, Smith and colleagues (1998) reported that the prevalence of BED among overweight participants in a population-based study was almost double (2.9%) that of the overall cohort (1.5%).

Age, Weight, Gender, and Ethnicity

With few exceptions (Bruce & Agras, 1992) most studies have found that obese subjects with BED seem to be significantly younger than non-binge-eating obese subjects, especially among obese patients presenting for treatment (e.g., de Zwaan et al., 1992). Compared to purging bulimics, however, obese binge eaters appear to be significantly older.

BED is associated with overweight and obesity, as evidenced by findings from clinic, community, and population-based studies (Wilfley et al., 2003).

Data indicate that BED is as common among black women as it is among white women—a relationship that appears to hold both within the community (Bruce & Agras, 1992; Striegel-Moore et al., 2000b; Striegel-Moore & Franko, 2003) and among those presenting for treatment (Yanovski et al., 1993, 1994). However, in a two-stage case-finding method, Striegel-Moore and colleagues (2003) found a significantly higher prevalence rate in white women (2.7%) compared to black women (1.4%) participating in the National Heart, Lung and Blood Institute Growth and Health Study. Nevertheless, relatively speaking, more women of minority race appear to meet criteria for BED than for BN. Race seems to play a role as well in the clinical presentation of BED. A study in a community sample of black and white women with BED found significant differences between the two groups. Black women with BED were heavier and reported more frequent binge eating; however, they reported less concern about body weight, shape, and eating and were less likely to have a history of BN than white women with BED (Pike et al., 2001). These results are consistent with survey studies that have shown that black women report less body image disturbance and are less likely to diet than white women (Smolak & Striegel-Moore, 2001). Cultural differences in the acceptance of larger body sizes might account for the lower level of disturbance in black women. Hispanic women appear to have comparable rates of binge eating to white women (Fitzgibbon et al., 1998); however, the prevalence of BED in Hispanic individuals is not known.

Available estimates are that women are roughly 1.5 times more likely to have BED than men (Spitzer et al., 1992, 1993b; Wilson et al., 1993). Thus, the gender imbalance concerning the prevalence of BED is less pronounced than in other eating disorders. Few studies have focused on gender differences in patients with BED (Barry et al., 2002; Lewinsohn et al., 2002; Striegel-Moore et al., 1998; Tanofsky et al., 1997). Men who experience problems with recurrent binge eating do not differ from female binge eaters on a wide range of indices of body image concerns, dieting behavior, and associated psychological distress. However, studies have found a significantly higher rate of substance abuse problems in men. There is also evidence that women struggle with more body image dissatisfaction and drive for thinness and are more likely to eat in response to negative emotions than men, whereas men are less likely to report distress over binge eating.

Binge Eating in Children and Adolescents

Decaluwe and colleagues (2002) administered the questionnaire version of the EDE (EDE-Q; Fairburn & Beglin, 1994) to 126 children and adolescents, ages 10–16 years old, who sought residential treatment for obesity. Binge-eating episodes were reported by 36.5% of the sample, with 6% reporting two or more episodes per week. Similar rates of binge-eating episodes were observed in boys and girls. As in adults, binge eaters reported more eating concerns, weight and shape concerns, and lower self-esteem. Applying the EDE interview, the same authors (Decaluwe & Breat, 2003) found a prevalence of BED of only 1% in a sample of 196 children and adolescents, ages 10–16 years, seeking weight loss treatment. Nine per cent were found to have objective bulimic episodes but did not endorse all of the DSM-IV criteria. The age of the first objective binge-eating episode was 10.8 years, and excessive weight gain appeared to precede binge eating. In a sample of 102 severely obese adolescents, ages 12–17 years, who were seeking treatment for their obesity, Isnard and colleagues (2003) assessed binge-eating symptoms using the Binge Eating Scale (BES; Gormally et al., 1982). They found three adolescent boys with severe binge-eating symptoms (≥ 26), and 16 (17%) adolescents (10 girls, 6 boys) with moderate to severe binge-eating symptoms (≥ 18).

Binge eaters were more depressed, more anxious, and had significantly lower self-esteem than non-binge eaters.

Lamerz and colleagues (2005) reported the results of 1,979 children, ages 5–6 years, who attended an obligatory health exam prior to school entry in Germany. The parents were asked to fill out questionnaires on their child's eating habits and weight development. The parents reported binge-eating episodes in 2% of their children, and there was a significant relationship between binge eating and obesity. In addition, binge eating in the children was strongly associated with eating disturbances in their mothers. In a school-based sample of adolescents, Ackard and colleagues (2003) found that 3.1% of the girls and 0.9% of the boys fulfilled DSM-IV criteria for BED. The available data suggest that clinically meaningful binge eating does occur in community samples and obese samples of children and adolescents. Dieting behavior may not be prominent in early-onset BED.

In order to adequately assess binge eating in children and adolescents, the interview and questionnaire versions of the EDE have been modified with simpler wording (ChEDE, ChEDE-Q; Bryant-Waugh et al., 1996).

It is unclear whether children have a full understanding of their eating behavior. In addition, children's access to food is usually more regulated by their parents. Many authors suggest that it may be appropriate to utilize broader and more flexible criteria that include developmentally appropriate aspects to screen children for eating disorders (Bryant-Waugh & Lask, 1995; Delacuwe et al., 2002; Marcus & Kalarchian, 2003; Nicholls et al., 2000). Eating disorders often present differently in children than they do in adults. Accordingly, modified criteria for BED in children and adolescents younger than 14 years of age have been proposed (Table 1.3; Marcus & Kalarchian, 2003). In children, eating in the absence of hunger, eating to modulate strong or negative affect, eating in secret, or hiding food may be correlates of binge eating. In addition, a shorter duration requirement (e.g., 3 months) might be more appropriate for children.

TABLE 1.3. Proposed BED Research Criteria for Children and Adolescents Younger Than 14 Years

A. Recurrent episodes of binge eating. An episode of binge eating is characterized by both of the following:
  (1) food seeking in the absence of hunger (e.g., after a full meal)
  (2) a sense of lack of control over eating (e.g., endorses "When I start to eat, I just can't stop")

B. The binge-eating episodes are associated with one or more of the following:
  (1) food seeking in response to negative affect (e.g., sadness, boredom, restlessness)
  (2) food seeking as a reward
  (3) sneaking or hiding food

C. Symptoms persist over a period of 3 months.

D. Eating is not associated with the regular use of inappropriate compensatory behaviors (e.g., purging, fasting, excessive exercise) and does not occur exclusively during the course of anorexia nervosa or bulimia nervosa.

Note. From Marcus and Kalarchian (2003). Copyright 2003 by Wiley Periodicals, Inc., A Wiley Company. Adapted by permission.

Summary

There is some evidence for the validity of BED as a diagnostic entity. Nevertheless, the current diagnostic criteria of BED, as they are outlined in the appendix of the DSM-IV, are still tentative, and alternative diagnostic classifications have been proposed. Studies evaluating new conceptualizations of BED are warranted. There is still much debate as to whether or not it is justified to give BED the status of a distinct diagnostic entity, and it is still unknown if the diagnosis will be included in DSM-V. Modified criteria for children and young adolescents have been proposed and should be evaluated, because binge eating usually begins at a young age and appears to be a prevalent problem even in children ages 5–6. The prevalence of BED in the general population is much higher compared to the prevalence of AN and BN, and the gender differences appear to be small. BED is a frequent phenomenon in treatment-seeking obese populations and needs to get proper attention from the health care professionals working with obese individuals. There is evidence that ethnically different groups are affected; however, most studies have been conducted with white females, and further studies will need to include male and ethnic minority groups. Finally, our knowledge about the psychosocial risk factors of BED is limited, and only prospective studies will help us gain more insight into these factors associated with the development of BED.

CHAPTER 2

Clinical Features, Longitudinal Course, and Psychopathology of Binge-Eating Disorder

Restraint/Dieting and Binge Eating in BED

In the BN literature, binge eating is often seen to develop in the context of dieting or restrained eating (Polivy & Herman, 1985). Restraint theory postulates that overeating results from the disruption of restraint in vulnerable individuals. In patients with BN, restrictive dieting is often viewed as a "precondition" for the development of binge eating and is central to most etiological and risk models. This factor also plays an important role in treatment approaches. However, the association between dieting/restraint and binge eating is less clear in individuals with BED.

First, scores on measures of dietary restraint (Three-Factor Eating Questionnaire [TFEQ], Stunkard & Messick, 1985; EDE, Fairburn & Cooper, 1993) are usually significantly lower in obese subjects with BED compared to patients with BN, and have shown either no correlation or even a negative correlation with binge eating among obese subjects (Brody et al., 1994; de Zwaan et al., 1994; Fichter et al., 1993; Kuehnel & Wadden, 1994; Lowe & Caputo, 1991; Marcus et al., 1985, 1992; Masheb & Grilo, 2000b, 2002; Molinari et al., 1997; Striegel-Moore et al., 2001; Wilfley et al., 2000a; Wilson et al., 1993). In parallel, laboratory studies have shown that subjects with BED consume more calories at both binge meals and nonbinge meals compared to weight-matched control participants without BED (e.g., Guss et al., 2002). Individuals with BN, on the other hand, consume more calories during a binge meal than do individuals with BED, but their caloric intake is far less during nonbinge meals (Mitchell et al., 1998).

Second, in BED, in contrast to BN, there is evidence that the onset of binge eating frequently occurs before the onset of self-reported dieting behavior, with at least 50% of patients developing binge eating in the absence of prior dieting in several studies (Tables 2.1 and 2.2).

TABLE 2.1. Sequence of Onset of Dieting and Binge Eating

Authors (year)	Diet-first	Binge-first	N, sample
Spitzer et al. (1993b)	37%	48.6%	387, weight control programs
Wilson et al. (1993)	8.7%	64%	37, weight-control program
Mussell et al. (1995)	25%	54.2%	30, clinical trial
Spurrell et al. (1997)	45%	55% (men 58%)	87, clinical trial
Abbott et al. (1998)	48.1%	38.7%	106, clinical trial
Grilo & Masheb (2000)	65%	35%	98, clinical trial
Manwaring et al. (2006)	19%	81%	155, New England Women's Health Project, community sample

TABLE 2.2. Differences between "Diet-First" and "Binge-First" Groups

	Authors (year)	Diet-first	Binge-first
Age first overweight (years)	Grilo & Masheb (2000)	15.8	12.4
	Marcus (1993)	18.0	13.0
	Marcus et al. (1995a)[a]	19.6	12.2
Age at onset of binge eating (years)	Manwaring et al. (2006)	24.5	19.1
	Grilo & Masheb (2000)	24.9	11.6
	Spurrell et al. (1997)	24.9	12.6
	Abbott et al. (1998)	25.7	11.8
	Marcus (1993)	24	13
	Marcus et al. (1995a)[a]	28.8	12.8
Age at onset of BED diagnosis (years)	Manwaring et al. (2006)	25.3	20.7
	Grilo & Masheb (2000)	25.8	17.8
	Spurrell et al. (1997)	33.2	18.8
Comorbidity	Manwaring et al. (2006) Abbott et al. (1998) Spurrell et al. (1997) Marcus (1993)	More substance use disorders	More psychiatric problems, more Axis II, more depression
Eating-related psychopathology	Manwaring et al. (2006)	More restraint and weight concerns	
Risk factors	Manwaring et al. (2006)	More repeated sexual abuse	More likely that someone close to them had died in the year before onset

[a]Early-onset versus late-onset group: onset of dieting 14.4 versus 20.4 years.

These "binge-first" groups are significantly younger at onset of binge eating, younger when first overweight, and younger at onset of meeting BED criteria compared to the "diet-first" groups. In addition, binge first groups have been found to report a higher frequency of weight-related teasing. In accordance with these results, women with early onset of BED (<18 years) were more likely than those with later onset of BED to binge-eat before dieting and to have early onset of obesity (Marcus et al., 1995a). Together, these findings strongly suggest that binge eating in younger children may not be coupled with efforts at dietary restriction. Because an early age of onset of binge eating has been shown to be related to poor treatment outcome, this finding is of considerable clinical importance (Agras et al., 1995; Safer et al., 2002). In the study by Agras and colleagues (1995), patients who reported that their binge-eating episodes began prior to age 16 were uniformly unsuccessful in treatment, whereas patients reporting that binge eating began after age 16 had a 75% success rate in a 24-week treatment program. This finding suggests the importance of early interventions for binge eating, prior to the onset of obesity. The binge-first groups also exhibited more eating-related psychopathology and were more likely to report a lifetime history of BN, mood disorders, and personality disorders (Abbott et al., 1998; Spurrell et al., 1997). However, in a recent community study Manwaring et al. (2006) failed to find more psychopathology in the binge-first group (81% of their sample) among women with BED. In this study the diet-first group was more likely to exhibit a lifetime diagnosis of substance use disorder and reported more eating-related psychopathology. In addition, the authors did not find significant differences in the overall prevalence of risk factors between binge-first and diet-first subtypes. An exploratory analysis of the Oxford Risk Factor Inventory (Fairburn et al., 1998) revealed that women in the binge-first group were more likely to have lost someone close to them in the year preceding binge-eating onset, and women in the diet-first group had experienced more sexual abuse.

Finally, weight loss treatments have not been shown to worsen binge eating among patients with BED, even though they usually increase restraint (Yanovski & Sebring, 1994; Yanovski et al., 1994). On the contrary, treatment studies for weight loss have generally reported significant reductions in binge eating, and subjects with BED are equally likely to report total adherence to weight loss programs, such as very-low-calorie diets (VLCDs), as non–binge eaters (de Zwaan et al., 2005b; LaPorte, 1992). It can be concluded that caloric restriction does not appear to be associated with the development of binge eating in individuals who have never reported problems with binge eating (Wadden et al., 2004a).

In summary, these two temporal patterns might provide meaningful subtypes of BED, raising the possibility of different etiological pathways for individuals with BED who report binge eating before dieting compared to those who report dieting first. It has been suggested that in BED binge eating might function to modulate negative emotional states, such as depression and anxiety, in patients who have made no previous attempt at dietary restriction (Agras & Telch, 1998; Binford et al., 2004). Masheb and Grilo (2006) reported that anxiety was the most frequently cited emotion leading to overeating in overweight patients with BED. This finding highlights the importance of examining functional aspects of binge eating with regard to affect regulation. Stice and Agras (1998) proposed a dual-pathway model of binge eating and suggested that body dissatisfaction is the key variable contributing to binge eating. In the restraint pathway model, body dissatisfaction accounts for restraint, which increases the likelihood of binge eating, and in the affect regulation pathway model, body dissatisfaction provokes negative affect, and binge eating is used to cope with negative affect by providing comfort and distraction.

Natural Course of BED

The natural course of BED remains controversial mainly because of variable results regarding the temporal stability and rates of spontaneous remission in those with BED. Cachelin and colleagues (1999) described the 6-month course of 31 individuals with BED in the community diagnosed with the EDE (Fairburn & Cooper, 1993). At the end of the 6 months, 10 of 31 subjects had been lost to follow-up. Of the remaining 21, 11 (52.4%) still met full BED criteria, whereas the other 10 were in partial remission. However, no subject was completely free of eating disorder symptoms at follow-up.

A larger community-based study investigated the 5-year course of 48 individuals with BED (Fairburn et al., 2000). Eight were lost to follow-up and of the remaining 40, only 7 (18%) had some form of clinical eating disorder after 5 years. This finding stands in contrast to those with BN, most of whom still met criteria for some form of clinically significant eating disorder after 5 years. This study provides evidence that BED might have a high spontaneous remission rate or may be an unstable state in which symptoms wax and wane. However, the sample investigated was relatively young (24.7 years) with a relatively low rate of obesity (21%). Subjects with BED gained, on average, 4.2 kg over the 5 years, and the percentage of subjects with a BMI of > 30 increased from 22 to 39%, indicating that BED may be a risk factor for future weight gain. In line with this observation, treatment studies with a no-treatment control group found that BED, if left untreated, leads to continued weight gain (Agras et al., 1995). In addition, follow-up results from BED treatment studies suggest that continued binge eating may be associated with a less favorable weight outcome (Agras et al., 1997; Raymond et al., 2002; Wilfley et al., 2002).

The largest community-based longitudinal study to date, funded by the McKnight Foundation, showed a much higher rate of diagnostic stability (Crow et al., 2002). This study examined the 4-year longitudinal course of individuals with AN, BN, and BED as well as with their subthreshold variants. The majority of the 104 individuals with BED (64%) had either full or subthreshold BED at the 1-year follow-up assessment and only 7% presented without any eating disorder diagnosis. For subthreshold BED a similar rate was seen (67%), with only 12% having no eating disorder diagnosis. At the 3-year assessment, 53% of individuals had cycled between BED and EDNOS. These data indicate that an eating disorder of clinical severity persists over a 3-year period in the majority of individuals suffering from full-syndrome BED. A preliminary analysis of the 4-year follow-up data shows that most individuals stayed within their initial broad diagnostic category. The frequencies of individuals without a diagnosable eating disorder at the 4-year follow-up were modest (for AN, 13%; for BN, 18%; for BED, 28%).

Fichter and colleagues (1998) reported the 3-, 6-, and 12-year course of 68 consecutively treated females with BED. At 6-year follow-up, the majority showed no major DSM-IV eating disorder: only 5.9% were still affected by full BED, 7.4% had shifted to BN purging type, 7.4% were classified as EDNOS, and one patient had died. At 12-year follow-up 7.8% still met criteria for BED, 9.4% had shifted to BN purging type, 12.5% were classified as EDNOS, and two patients (3.2%) had died. More than 67% did not have an eating disorder as defined by the DSM-IV. Interestingly, the course of BED was very similar to BN, and psychiatric comorbidity was a robust predictor of an unfavorable course for both disorders (Fichter & Quadflieg, 2005).

Recently, Wade and colleagues (2006) reported that 3 of 29 women (10%) with a lifetime history of BED still exhibited full diagnostic criteria for BED at the time of the interview, which was conducted, on average, 13.5 years after initial onset of objective binge eating. Ten were classified as asymptomatic (34.5%) and 10 as having a good outcome (69% combined). Interestingly, these percentages were lower compared to women with a history of AN or BN, where at minimum, good outcome was achieved by 84% and 76%, respectively. Overall, outcome was relatively good; however, less than 50% of any eating-disordered group was asymptomatic at the time of the interview.

As opposed to natural course studies, there is evidence from retrospective community studies and from treatment-seeking samples that BED is a stable and persistent disorder (Pope et al., 2006; Wilfley et al., 2003). Mussell and colleagues (1995) reported that the mean age at which participants presented for treatment was 45 years, with an onset of the syndrome 20 years earlier. However, the treatment literature indicates that most of the proposed treatments for BED result in significant improvement in binge-eating symptoms or remission of the disorder. This finding may also be consistent with a high spontaneous remission rate or a high response rate to nonspecific treatment modalities.

Eating-Related Psychopathology

Reviews of the literature suggest that obese individuals with BED differ significantly from obese individuals without BED in several important ways, including an early-age onset of obesity, a higher percentage of reported time on diets, and more frequent weight fluctuations (Brody et al., 1994; de Zwaan et al., 1994; Yanovski et al., 1994). BED patients are significantly and meaningfully different from overweight and normal-weight control subjects without BED in many of the dimensions of eating psychopathology. Moreover, the association of BED with obesity becomes stronger with increasing levels of BMI (Hudson et al., 2006). Patients with BED are very similar to patients with AN and BN in terms of their level of dysfunctional attitudes regarding eating and overvalued ideas regarding weight and shape. Subjects with BED reported significantly increased attitudinal disturbance in body dissatisfaction and size perception compared to subjects without BED (Mussell et al., 1996a). This correlation has been found in clinical as well as community samples and is not explained by the degree of depression (Barry et al., 2003; Masheb & Grilo, 2000a; Striegel-Moore et al., 2001). Moreover, the majority of treatment-seeking patients with BED reported regularly pinching areas of their body to check for fatness and avoiding clothes that made them particularly aware of their body (Reas et al., 2005). These results suggest that dysfunctional attitudes regarding eating, weight, and shape reflect the core eating disorder psychopathology not only of BN but also of BED. These symptoms might therefore be included as diagnostic features of BED because they might have implications for treatment (Eldredge & Agras, 1996; Masheb & Grilo, 2000a; Striegel-Moore et al., 1998, 2001; Wilfley et al., 2000a;). When the effects of age and depression levels are controlled, treatment-seeking women with BN are generally similar to those with BED (Barry et al., 2003). The primary difference between individuals with BED and those with AN and BN is that obese individuals with BED usually exhibit significantly lower eating restraint scores. Extreme dietary restraint is part of the characteristic psychopathology for patients with AN or BN, but this is not the case for patients with BED. In addition, there is usually no difference in levels of restraint between obese individuals with and without BED (Wilfley et al., 2000c).

Mitchell and colleagues (1999) investigated the hedonics of binge eating in treatment-seeking women with BED or BN. Subjects with BED were more likely to report that they enjoyed the food—its taste, smell, and texture—while binge eating. In addition, the BED group reported more relaxation and less physical discomfort and anxiety as a consequence of binge eating compared to the BN group.

How to address the eating patterns and problematic eating behavior in those with BED is addressed in Part II of this book, which includes a detailed treatment manual. Some of the treatment overlaps with the cognitive-behavioral therapy (CBT) used for BN, but some is unique to BED.

General Psychopathology

In clinical samples as well as in community samples, most investigations have found significantly higher levels of general psychopathology in obese patients with BED than in those without binge eating (Antony et al., 1994; Brody et al., 1994; Fichter et al., 1993; Marcus et al., 1988; Schlundt et al., 1991; Spitzer et al., 1993b; Striegel-Moore et al., 1998) but significantly lower levels compared to patients with BN (Brody et al., 1994; Fichter et al., 1993; Raymond et al., 1995; Spitzer et al., 1993b). This psychopathology includes higher depression and anxiety scores, a higher frequency of negative automatic thoughts, a higher frequency of past psychotherapeutic contact, an increased prevalence of impulsive behaviors, and higher anger levels (Bulik et al., 2002; Fassino et al., 2003). Obese patients with BED also report significantly lower self-esteem (de Zwaan et al., 1994; Lowe & Caputo 1991; Striegel-Moore et al., 1998) and lower self-efficacy (Miller et al., 1999) than non–binge eaters.

Several studies have assessed alexithymia in obese patients with BED. The term *alexithymia* is used to describe a personality trait characterized by the inability to experience and express emotions. Alexithymia was elevated in some (Pinaquy et al., 2003) but not all studies (de Zwaan et al., 1995) in patients with BED. However, there appears to be a relationship between emotional eating and alexithymic personality traits, which has shown to be stronger in obese men than women (Larsen et al., 2006; Pinaquy et al., 2003).

Health-related and weight-related quality of life have consistently been shown to be more impaired in obese individuals with BED compared to obese individuals without BED (de Zwaan et al., 2003a; Kolotkin et al., 2004; Rieger et al., 2005).

Psychiatric Comorbidity

Individuals with BED have significantly higher rates of lifetime Axis I comorbidity compared to obese individuals without BED. Prevalence rates have ranged from 42 to 81% for any diagnosis in various treatment-seeking and non-treatment-seeking BED samples. For example, relative to an overweight non-eating-disordered sample, individuals who suffered from BED were three times more likely to suffer from current major depression, with lifetime prevalence rates ranging from 32 to 91% (Bulik et al., 2002; Hudson et al., 1988; LaPorte, 1992; Marcus et al., 1988, 1990a; Mussell et al., 1996b; Specker et al., 1994; Spitzer et al., 1993b; Telch & Stice, 1998; Wilfley et al., 2000a, 2000c; Yanovski et al., 1993). The results of controlled studies are summarized in Tables 2.3, 2.4, and 2.5.

TABLE 2.3. Lifetime Prevalence Rates in Percentage of Axis I Disorders, Using Structured Clinical Interviews in Treatment-Seeking Samples of Obese Binge Eaters and Non–Binge Eaters

Authors (year)	Sample size	Diagnostic criteria	Any Axis I diagnosis	Any affective disorder	Major depression	Substance use disorder	Anxiety disorder	BN
Hudson et al. (1988)								
BE	23	Obese bulimia (DSM-III)	—	91[a]	87[a] 21	17	—	
Non-BE	47	obesity	—	45	40	15	13	—
Marcus et al. (1990a)								
BE	25	BES ≥29	60[a]	32[a]	24	12	20	—
Non-BE	25	Obesity	28	8	4	4	12	—
Yanovski et al. (1993)								
BED	43	DSM-IV	60[a]	—	51[a]	12	9 (panic)[a]	7[a]
Non-BED	85	Obesity	34	—	14	8	1	0
Brody et al. (1994)								
BED	13	DSM-IV	41.7	33.3	—	8.3	—	—
Non-BED	54		24	17	—	13	—	—
Specker et al. (1994)								
BED	43	DSM-IV	72.1[a]	48.8[a]	47[a]	27.9	11.6	18.6[a]
Non-BED	57	Obesity	49.1	29.5	26.3	22.8	10.5	0
Mussell et al. (1996b)								
BED	80	DSM-IV	70[a]	50[a]	46.3[a]	22.5[a]	18.8	12.5[a]
Non-BED	48	Obesity	29.2	19.8	18.8	4.2	10.4	0

Note: BN, bulimia nervosa; BE, binge eaters; BED, binge-eating disorder; BES, Binge Eating Scale.
[a]Significant difference.

TABLE 2.4. Lifetime Prevalence Rates in Percentage of Axis I Disorders, Using Structured Clinical Interviews in Community Samples

Authors (year)	BED (n)	Diagnostic criteria	Any Axis I diagnosis	Any affective disorder	Major depression	Substance use disorder	Anxiety disorder	BN
Telch & Stice (1998)								
BED	61	DSM-IV	59[a]	—	49[a]	15 (alcohol)	12 (panic)	2
Non-BED	60		37	—	28	10	7	0
Bulik et al. (2002)								
Obese BE[c]	59	Binge eating	—	—	47.5[a]	17.0 (alcohol)[a]	25.4[a]	—
Obese Non-BE	107		—	—	26.2	5.6	(panic[b]) 7.5	—

Note. BN, bulimia nervosa; BED, binge-eating disorder; BE, binge eaters.
[a]Significantly higher values compared to control group.
[b]Broadly defined.
[c]Nonbulimic.

The increased psychiatric comorbidity among individuals with BED appears to be attributable to the severity of binge eating rather than the degree of obesity. Depressive symptomatology may render individuals more vulnerable to binge-eating relapse, and binge eating might be used as a means to regulate affect (Mussell et al., 1995; Telch & Stice, 1998). There is some evidence that BED frequently predates the development of affective symptoms (Mussell et al., 1995), suggesting that depression might be a consequence of this eating disorder. However, the sequence of binge-eating onset and psychiatric comorbidity as well as the causality of the comorbidity require further study. Because comorbid depression is more the norm than the ex-

TABLE 2.5. Lifetime Prevalence Rates in Percentage of Axis I Disorders, Using Structured Clinical Interviews in Treatment-Seeking BED Samples Compared to Non-Treatment-Seeking BED Samples and Psychiatric Controls

Authors (year)	BED (n)	Diagnostic criteria	Any Axis I diagnosis	Any affective disorder	Major depression	Substance use disorder	Anxiety disorder	BN
Wilfley et al. (2000a)								
BED treatment	162	DSM-IV	77	61	58	23	13	—
Psychiatric samples[a]	—		—		40	26 (alcohol)	15 (panic)	—
Wilfley et al. (2001)								
BED treatment	37	DSM-IV	81	68	—	50	22	—
BED community	108		81	63	—	42	39	—

Note. BN, bulimia nervosa; BED, binge-eating disorder.
[a]From First et al. (1995) and Williams et al. (1992).

ception in patients with BED, this comorbidity might have implications for treatment. However, Wilfley and colleagues (2000a) did not find an influence of any specific area of Axis I comorbidity on treatment outcome in patients with BED participating in group CBT or interpersonal therapy (IPT).

The findings concerning anxiety disorders and substance abuse are controversial. One study found higher rates of panic disorder (Yanovski et al., 1993) in obese subjects with, compared to those without, BED. Only one study found higher rates of substance abuse (Mussell et al., 1996a) in obese subjects with BED compared to subjects without BED.

Of note, eating, mood, and anxiety disorders have shown to aggregate in the families of women with BED compared to women without BED (Fairburn et al., 1998; Fowler & Bulik, 1997; Striegel-Moore et al., 2002).

A history of AN seems to be very rare (McCann et al., 1991; Specker et al., 1994); a history of BN, on the other hand, seems to be more common in patients with BED than in those without BED, with prevalence rates ranging between 7 and 29% in treatment-seeking samples (Mussell et al., 1996a; Specker et al., 1994; Yanovski et al., 1993) and 2 to 10% in community samples (Striegel-Moore et al., 2001; Telch & Stice, 1998). Overall, these findings suggest that BED, in most cases, does not seem to present a "burned out" form of BN. In addition, a history of BN in subjects with BED does not appear to be associated with increased rates of comorbid psychopathology, severity of eating problems, dietary restraint, or attitudinal disturbance (Peterson et al., 1998).

Community Samples

In a population-based sample, binge eating was associated with a significantly increased risk for lifetime major depression, panic disorder, any phobia, or alcohol dependence (Bulik et al., 2002). Telch and Stice (1998) found fewer differences in rates of current and lifetime comorbid psychiatric disorders between women with BED and those without BED in the community. However, they too found a significantly higher lifetime prevalence rate of major depression in the sample of women with BED.

It is well known that people with more than one type of psychiatric problem are more likely to seek treatment than those with only one problem (Berkson's bias [1946]), resulting in an overestimation of comorbidity in clinical samples. However, Wilfley et al. (2001) did not find any differences in current and lifetime prevalence rates of psychiatric diagnoses between a clinic sample of 37 patients with BED and 108 community cases of BED. Interestingly, Wilfley and colleagues (2001) reported that community BED cases were over nine times more likely to have a current anxiety disorder than treatment-seeking cases (20% vs. 3%), suggesting that comorbid anxiety problems may inhibit treatment seeking among individuals with BED. These results suggest that studies using treatment-seeking samples may not have overestimated the rate of comorbid psychiatric disorders. Clinical samples show, however, a more severe eating disorder and a higher level of social impairment (Wilfley et al., 2001), suggesting the presence of more personality disturbance and lack of social support.

Comparison between BED and BN

Comparisons between patients with BED and those with BN present a somewhat mixed picture. Significantly higher current and lifetime prevalence rates of affective disorders are seen in patients with BN when compared with nonpurging BN patients and obese binge eaters (McCann et al., 1991; Raymond et al., 1995; Spitzer et al., 1993b). However, other studies found similar prevalence rates of affective disorders in subjects with BED or BN (Alger et al., 1991; Fichter et al., 1993; Hudson et al., 1988; Schwalberg et al., 1992). Also, in community samples comorbidity rates did not differ between women with BED, purging BN, and nonpurging BN (Striegel-Moore et al., 2001).

Personality Disorders

Although fewer studies have examined the pattern of Axis II diagnoses associated with BED, they have consistently found higher prevalence rates of these disorders among BED than non-BED obese samples in treatment-seeking as well as community contexts (Cassin & von Ranson, 2005; Specker et al., 1994; Telch & Stice, 1998; van Hanswijck de Jonge, 2003; Wilfley et al., 2000a; Yanovski et al., 1993), with rates ranging from 20 to 37%. These studies suggest that avoidant, obsessive–compulsive, and borderline personality disorders are the most common Axis II disorders in those with BED. Axis II psychopathology was significantly related to severity of binge eating and eating-related psychopathology at baseline, and Cluster B personality disorder was related to outcome, predicting significantly higher levels of binge eating at 1-year follow-up after group CBT or IPT (Wilfley et al., 2000a). This finding accords with other findings in patients with BN.

Summary

Obese individuals with BED are different from obese individuals without BED and show many similarities to those with BN regarding eating-related and general psychopathology as well as Axis I and Axis II psychiatric comorbidity. There are, however, several differences. Individuals with BED have a low risk of AN and show less restraint over eating compared to those with BN. In BED dietary restraint appears to be unrelated to binge-eating frequency. In about half of the cases the onset of binge eating occurs in the absence of dieting, which stands in contrast to BN and suggests that binge eating, in BED, might be precipitated more frequently by adverse affective experiences.

The natural course of BED is controversial mainly because of conflicting results regarding stability and rates of spontaneous remission of the disorder. Some prospective studies show persistence of BED symptomatology, whereas others suggest a tendency to remit over time. The heterogeneity of results may be due to differences in age and duration of illness in the populations assessed. In clinical settings patients with BED usually report a long history of the disorder.

CHAPTER 3

Binge-Eating Disorder and Obesity

Although it is clear that binge eating can occur in normal weight and even underweight individuals, the relative rarity with which nonoverweight individuals present for treatment for BED, as reflected in the paucity of available information (see Chapters 6 and 7), suggests that the association of binge eating and obesity has, at a minimum, important clinical significance. A relationship between overweight/obesity and binge eating has been demonstrated in nonclinical samples as well, both within (French et al., 1999) and outside the United States (Siqueira et al., 2004). Much less clear is the *nature* of the relationship between BED and obesity, particularly the etiological and pathophysiological underpinnings of the observed association. This chapter attempts to pose and answer, to the degree possible based on current knowledge, some of the most interesting and important questions concerning this relationship.

Is Obesity an Eating Disorder in and of Itself?

Before considering the relationship between BED and obesity per se, an even more basic question merits consideration: Is obesity, in and of itself, properly considered an eating disorder—that is, a subcategory of mental disorders? If so, then the designation of BED for an obese individual would serve as a specifier of the type of disordered eating she/he manifests, and the distinction between obese BED and obese non-BED would be much less significant.

According to DSM-IV, a mental disorder is "a clinically significant behavioral or psychological syndrome or pattern that occurs in an individual and that is associated with present distress (e.g., a painful symptom) or disability (i.e., impairment in one or more important areas of functioning) or with a significantly increased risk of suffering death, pain, disability, or an important loss of freedom. . . . Whatever its cause, it must currently be considered a manifestation of a behavioral, psychological, or biological dysfunction in the individual" (American Psychiatric Association, 2000a, p. xxxi).

In order for the diagnosis of obesity to fit this definition, those characterized as obese would have to (1) manifest abnormal behavioral or psychological features and (2) suffer from distress, disability, or an increased risk of morbidity or mortality. Is the eating behavior of obese individuals abnormal? Although early studies relying on self-report suggested that obese individuals do not eat more than those of normal weight, doubly labeled water studies, using a highly accurate method for assessing total energy expenditure (Schoeller et al., 1986), have demonstrated that obese individuals do indeed eat more than their normal-weight counterparts (Black et al., 1993). However, it has been argued that because obese individuals eat an appropriate amount to maintain their larger body size—that is, their normalized total energy expenditure is not different from normal-weight individuals (Schutz & Jequier, 2004)—this difference ought not to be considered pathological (Devlin et al., 2000). In addition, even regular consumption of unusually large meals would not, in and of itself, meet the definition of an eating binge, which also requires the experience of loss of control. This distinction is a significant one; when loss of control is added into the definition of an eating binge, the proportion of obese individuals who qualify as binge eaters is greatly reduced (Spitzer et al., 1992).

Do obese individuals suffer from distress, disability, or increased medical risk? Despite the multiple manifestations of obesity-related stigma in our culture, including discrimination in employment, health care, and education (Puhl & Brownell, 2001), obese individuals vary widely in their degree of obesity-related distress (Heinberg et al., 2001), and distress is not a universal concomitant of obesity. Regarding disability and medical risk, the significant morbidity and mortality related to obesity are well known and have been thoroughly reviewed (Fontaine & Allison, 2004; Manson et al., 2004). Yet medical fitness can be improved even without significant weight loss, and disease risk may be related to lifestyle and other variables more so than body weight or body composition per se (Miller, 1999).

Obesity-related disability may also occur in the psychological and/or cognitive realms. Most studies of psychiatric comorbidity in obese samples suggest that clinical but not community samples of the obese show increased psychiatric disorder rates (Wadden et al., 2002). However, recent community epidemiological studies have shown a small increase in depression risk in severely obese women (Onyike et al., 2003). Few studies have rigorously assessed the impact of obesity on cognitive function, but there are hints that obesity may be associated with impaired performance on various cognitive tests (Jeong et al., 2005; Kilander et al., 1997), although the mechanism of this association is unclear. Finally, a fairly robust literature suggests that obesity is related to impairments in health-related quality of life in both physical and mental health domains (Wadden et al., 2002).

In sum, although the case for obesity-associated disability and/or risk in at least some obese individuals is strong, the lack of a universal obesity-related abnormality in behavior or psychological features argues against the concept of obesity as primarily a mental disorder. However, the presence of prominent obesity-associated disabilities in several realms leaves the door open to considering subpopulations, such as individuals with BED who do have clear disturbances in eating behavior and often in psychological function, as suffering from a mental disorder, specifically an eating disorder. And the relationship between some of the clinical features of BED (see Chapter 2) and those of the classical eating disorders of AN and BN provides further support for the idea of BED as an eating disorder that occurs primarily, at least in clinical populations, in the obese. It is important to note that even "non-normative" eating patterns that do not meet the threshold for mental disorders may have a significant impact on weight, adiposity, and overall health (Tanofsky-Kraff & Yanovski, 2004).

How Frequently Do BED and Obesity Coexist?

The percentage of obese individuals who suffer from BED varies greatly depending on the nature of the sample and the method used to diagnose BED. Several early studies (e.g., Spitzer et al., 1992, 1993b) using self-report methods found prevalences of BED as high as 20–30% in weight control samples as opposed to rates of 2–3% in mostly normal-weight community samples. However, interview-based studies have reported significantly lower rates of BED in both types of samples, with rates as low as 1% in the general population and less than 5% in obesity treatment samples, although as many as 10–25% in weight loss samples report binge eating that does not meet formal criteria for BED (Williamson & Martin, 1999). In epidemiological community samples, studies using both self-report (Smith et al., 1998) and interview methods (Hay, 1998; Kinzl et al., 1999) have consistently demonstrated an association between BED and weight, with rates of binge eating in overweight and obese subjects at least double those in normal-weight individuals. Within the obese, it has long been known that rates of binge eating increase with increasing adiposity (Telch et al., 1988). Moreover, BED seems to be associated with early onset of obesity (Mussell et al., 1995).

Looking at the question of BED–obesity overlap from the other direction—that is, the percentage of individuals with BED who are obese—is also of interest. Here there is clearly an important selection bias in clinical studies. Most clinics that treat individuals with BED report that these individuals have varying degrees of obesity and typically have long histories of repeated dieting (American Psychiatric Association, 2000, p. 786). Indeed, most clinical studies of BED include chiefly or exclusively overweight individuals. Yet community-based studies suggest that there are far more normal-weight binge eaters than one would imagine from the clinical literature. As recently summarized by Didie and Fitzgibbon (2005), in community- and clinic-based samples without weight restrictions, nearly half of individuals who meet criteria for BED are not even overweight. This discrepancy between the large number of normal-weight individuals with BED and their minimal representation in clinical trials for BED raises several interesting possibilities. One possibility is that normal-weight individuals with BED are not sufficiently distressed to seek treatment or do not consider their binge eating a reason to seek treatment. Another possibility is that these individuals are interested in treatment, but that the perceived or actual availability of treatment for BED in the absence of obesity is limited. Further attention to the needs of normal-weight individuals with BED is very much needed.

What Is the Central Clinical Feature of Obese Binge Eaters?

Obese individuals with BED present a challenge for clinicians and nosologists alike, in part because their disorder is not limited to a single dimension. In fact, such individuals suffer from a constellation of difficulties that includes *physiological* (i.e., obesity), *behavioral* (i.e., binge eating), and *psychological* (i.e., distress related to body shape and weight, frequent comorbid psychopathology) aspects. Depending on what is identified as the central clinical feature of BED, the approach to treatment and the evaluation of the treatment outcome may vary greatly. If the emphasis is placed on obesity and binge eating is seen merely as a means of becoming or remaining obese, then treatment must address weight, and any treatments that did not yield significant weight loss would be seen as ineffective. Likewise, theoretical emphases on the behavior of binge eating or on the psychological distress associated with BED carry with them their own very practical implications for treatment and the evaluation of treatment outcome.

The various theoretical models of BED have been reviewed in detail elsewhere (Devlin et al., 2003) and are summarized in Figure 3.1. Models 1 and 2 emphasize binge eating and do not require the presence of obesity. Models 3 and 4 are particularly relevant to the topic of obesity and BED, because both include obesity as an explicit feature of the syndrome. Model 3 views BED as a potentially meaningful behavioral subtype of obesity, relegating binge eating to the role of a behavioral pattern that contributes to the onset or maintenance of an overweight state. Evidence suggesting that binge eating does indeed contribute to obesity is summarized below (Question 4). However, there is little evidence that the successful treatment of binge eating brings about significant weight loss (although it may mitigate further weight gain) or that obese binge eaters who are primarily seeking treatment for obesity should receive different treatment than obese nonbinge eaters with the same goal (Devlin et al., 2003). In light of such evidence, it is difficult to make a strong case for BED as a clinically useful behavioral subtype of obesity at this point. However, to the degree to which binge eating contributes to the onset of obesity, the timely identification and treatment of binge eating could play an important role in the *prevention* of obesity, even if it is not an important factor in the *treatment* of established obesity. In addition, it is clear that obese individuals with BED differ from equally obese individuals without BED in a variety of ways, including both psychological and behavioral features (see Chap-

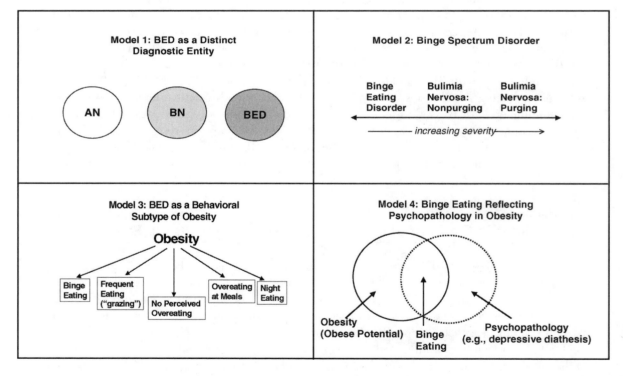

FIGURE 3.1. Models of BED. From Devlin, Goldfein, and Dobrow (2003). Copyright 2003 by Wiley Periodicals, Inc., A Wiley Company. Adapted by permission.

ters 2 and 5); what is less clear is the relevance of these differences to the onset or maintenance of obesity.

Model 4 views binge eating as an epiphenomenon that emerges when obesity or obese potential overlaps with a psychological feature such as a depressive diathesis, an impulsive temperament, or significant distress related to body shape or weight. Under such circumstances, according to this model, an individual may develop binge eating—which, however, is not so much a problem in its own right as it is a reflection of a deeper problem. The implication for treatment is that the more appropriate focus would be the underlying problems (obesity, psychological features), not the symptom (binge eating). Circumstantial evidence supporting various versions of this model has been reviewed elsewhere (Devlin et al., 2003). However, a more definitive approach would be to study longitudinally the cluster of obesity and binge eating, on one hand, and the cluster of obesity and psychopathology, on the other, and determine the relative stability over time, association with course of obesity, and clinical utility (e.g., reliable association with clinical factors such as quality of life or health care utilization) of the two competing syndrome definitions. Studies suggesting that dysphoria and depression may be mediating factors in the relationship between binge eating status and weight loss success (Linde et al., 2004; Sherwood et al., 1999) begin to provide the sort of evidence that is needed to answer this question.

In considering the relationship of obesity with BED, studies examining the differences between obese and nonobese individuals with BED are particularly relevant. Despite the potential importance of this distinction in rethinking diagnostic criteria, particularly the question of whether the diagnosis should require obesity or overweight, relatively few studies have rigorously compared these groups. Studies of individuals seeking treatment for BED have reported no differences in psychological or eating symptom measures between obese and nonobese subjects (Didie & Fitzgibbon, 2005) or only minimal differences between the two groups (Barry et al., 2003). A large-scale study of nonclinical women enrolled in a weight gain prevention program similarly found that binge eating had similar correlates (dieting, depression, weight/shape preoccupation) in normal-weight and overweight women. Consistent with this finding, most studies examining the relationship between level of obesity and clinical features in subjects with and without binge eating have reported that presence/absence of binge eating, but not severity of obesity, is associated with comorbid psychopathology (Picot & Lilenfeld, 2003; Yanovski et al., 1993). In addition, in a mixed-weight sample of individuals with and without binge eating, binge eating was found to be associated with abdominal pain and dyschezia, regardless of weight. Obesity was found to be associated with constipation, diarrhea, straining, and flatus (Crowell et al., 1994). Thus, despite their relative absence in clinical trials, there is little support for excluding individuals from the BED diagnostic category on the basis of weight. However, it is the case that obese individuals with BED manifest an additional aspect in their clinical presentation that has its own associated morbidity and presents an additional potential target for treatment.

Does Binge Eating Cause or Result from Obesity?

As discussed above, very different models of BED have been proposed with different etiological underpinnings and different implications for treatment. One model of etiology suggests that binge eating may lead to the onset or persistence of obesity. Another suggests that dieting in

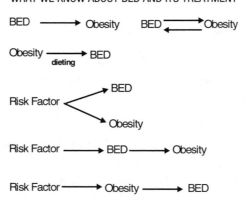

FIGURE 3.2. Possible causal relationships between BED and obesity.

response to actual or perceived overweight may lead to the emergence of binge eating. And, of course, it is possible that both relationships exist, creating a positive feedback loop in which binge eating and obesity are mutually promoting. Additionally, it is possible that neither causal relationship exists, but rather that a common risk factor or set of risk factors accounts for the frequent association of binge eating and obesity. In fact, as has been suggested in retrospective community-based studies of risk factors, it is likely that there are multiple risk factors for BED, some of which also confer risk for obesity and others of which do not (Fairburn et al., 1998). Figure 3.2 summarizes these varying causal relationships.

Evidence of Binge Eating Leading to Obesity

One of the early studies suggesting a causal relationship between binge eating and obesity was the 5-year longitudinal study by Fairburn and colleagues (2000) of young women in the community with BED. At the final follow-up point, the prevalence of obesity had, strikingly, nearly doubled, although most subjects no longer met criteria for BED. A more recent prospective community-based cohort study of young adults followed over a period of 20 years from ages 19 to 40 found that binge eating was associated with both being overweight and with increased weight gain over time (Hasler et al., 2004). Other longitudinal studies reporting an association between binge eating and subsequent weight gain and/or obesity onset include a 4-year study of Northern California female high school students, which found that both dieting and binge eating predicted greater than expected weight gain over time (Stice et al., 1999); a 2-year prospective investigation of adolescent girls, which found that the frequency of binge eating at the beginning of the study predicted the onset of obesity during the study period (Stice et al., 2002); a 3-year longitudinal study of children ages 9–14, which found an association in boys but not girls between binge eating and weight gain (Field et al., 2003); and a recent 4-year study of children ages 6–12, which found that binge eating predicted increases in body fat over time (Tanofsky-Kraff et al., 2006). However, in a recent study of adolescent girls ages 11–15 followed over 4 years, Stice and colleagues (2005) did not detect a relationship between binge eating and the onset of obesity. Nonetheless, the weight of the evidence from longitudinal studies suggests that binge eating may indeed promote excessive weight gain and obesity.

Another line of evidence supporting the suggestion that binge eating contributes to obesity comes from treatment studies of obese individuals with binge eating. Several such studies (Agras et al., 1997; Raymond et al., 2002; Sherwood et al., 1999; Wilfley et al., 2002) have noted that binge cessation was associated with relative weight stability over time, compared to ongoing weight gain in individuals who continued to binge eat. Similarly, McGuire and colleagues (1999), using data from the National Weight Control Registry of successful weight loss maintainers, found that binge eating at entry into the registry predicted weight regain.

Although it seems likely that binge eating does indeed promote weight gain and the development of obesity, the mechanism by which binge eating produces this effect is somewhat less clear. As reviewed elsewhere in this volume (see Chapter 5), a number of studies has reported that obese individuals with BED, compared to equally obese non–binge eaters, consume more in a laboratory meal whether instructed to binge eat or to eat normally without binge eating. This finding suggests that individuals with BED may simply be in a state of positive energy balance (i.e., caloric intake exceeding caloric expenditure)—which, by the law of energy conservation, must lead to weight gain over time. However, it may not be the case that consumption of a single meal in a laboratory accurately reflects overall intake. Alger and colleagues (1995) studied obese binge eaters and non-bingers in a respiratory chamber, in which daily intake, total energy expenditure, and components of energy expenditure were measured, and found similar mean daily energy intake in the two groups, with greater day-to-day variability in intake among binge eaters. Consistent with this finding, a study using a rigorous dietary recall methodology found no difference in overall daily intake between obese subjects with and without BED, but considerable difference in eating by subjects with BED on binge versus non-binge days (Raymond et al., 2003).

Another possible mechanism by which binge eating might lead to the development of excess weight or obesity rests on the idea that the intermittent dieting and weight gain cycling that is characteristic of individuals with BED may have physiological effects that promote metabolic efficiency and weight gain. However, the idea that weight cycling promotes weight gain over time has not been borne out clearly (Hill, 2004). A related concept is that a pattern of binge eating alternating with strict control of eating, such as that seen in BN, may promote weight gain over time. Although also controversial, this argument is probably moot in the case of BED because, as several studies have suggested, in contrast to the feast-or-famine pattern seen in BN, individuals with BED tend to overeat throughout the day (Marcus et al., 1992; Yanovski & Sebring, 1994).

Investigations on the psychobiology of binge eating have suggested that there are physiological abnormalities, such as increased gastric capacity and abnormalities in fasting and postprandial ghrelin (Geliebter et al., 2004b, 2005), that may conceivably result from binge eating and contribute to subsequent weight gain—although this relationship has yet to be demonstrated. Consistent with this idea, though, is the finding that baseline and postprandial ghrelin tend to become more normal following binge cessation (Geliebter et al., 2005). Another line of research that suggests a possible link between binge eating and the development of obesity involves the stress response in obese subjects with BED. Gluck reported that obese subjects with BED, compared to obese subjects without BED, reported exaggerated stress responses, as manifested by increased levels of hunger and desire to binge eat following stress induction (cold pressor test), and also that cortisol stress response is correlated with central obesity in obese women with BED (Gluck, 2006). Taken together, these findings begin to make a case for some aspect of BED, perhaps the associated exaggerated stress reactivity, contributing to subsequent obesity. Further research in this area is greatly needed.

Evidence of Obesity Leading to Binge Eating

The most common theoretical argument in favor of a causal pathway from obesity to BED invokes dieting or dietary restraint as a mediator between obesity and binge eating. In other words, individuals who are obese or at risk for becoming obese might initiate dieting as an attempt to control their weight and then subsequently develop binge eating. The widely accepted cognitive-behavioral model of binge eating, originally developed to describe the maintenance of binge eating and vomiting in individuals with BN, suggests that binge eating is a response to overly rigid control of eating, which periodically gives way to episodes of uncontrolled eating. The application of this model to binge eating is somewhat complex, however, because binge eating in obese patients does not, for the most part, result from dietary restraint as it is usually understood, and a substantial proportion of patients with BED begin binge eating before the onset of dieting (de Zwaan, 2001). However, several studies do suggest an association between dieting and binge eating in children ages 10–16 (Decaluwe & Braet, 2005), adolescents (Ackard et al., 2003), and adults (Polivy, 1996). Moreover, as previously mentioned, a community-based study of risk factors found that obesity-related risk factors were predictive of BED, although this relationship was less pronounced than the relationship between obesity-related risk factors and BN (Fairburn et al., 1998).

However, in a clinical context, the relationship between dieting as a treatment for obesity and binge eating may be very different. A substantial literature on the use of very-low-calorie diets in individuals with BED suggests that, although a small number may develop breakthrough binge eating (Yanovski et al., 1994), most do not (Wonderlich et al., 2003). And, in an important recent report, it was conclusively demonstrated that a low-calorie dieting program for obese non–binge eaters did not lead to the *de novo* emergence of binge eating (Wadden et al., 2004). It remains to be investigated whether this is equally true in obese individuals with a past history of binge eating. Thus, the causal relationship between obesity, dieting, and the onset of binge eating in community samples, to the degree to which it does indeed exist, might have relatively few implications for treatment (see Question 5).

Another way in which obesity might increase the risk for BED is via obesity-associated distress. There is substantial evidence that obesity is associated with significant stigma (Puhl & Brownell, 2001), and certainly chronic stigmatization can be associated with significant distress for most individuals. It is well known that distress increases eating in chronic dieters, that most obese individuals tend to be dieters, and that obese individuals overeat relative to normal-weight individuals when stressed (Polivy & Herman, 1999). The binge-promoting effect of negative affect in obese women with BED has been demonstrated in the laboratory (Agras & Telch, 1998). It therefore seems likely that obesity-associated distress may help to maintain binge eating in obese individuals; that it promotes the onset of BED is plausible but has yet to be convincingly demonstrated.

Evidence of Common Risk Factors for Binge Eating and Obesity

The genetic risk factors for BED have been reviewed elsewhere in this volume (see Chapter 4), including the putative (Branson et al., 2003) and now controversial (Hebebrand et al., 2004; Lubrano-Berthelier et al., 2006) association between mutations in the melanocortin-4 receptor, a known cause of childhood-onset obesity, and binge eating in obese adults. However, even if such an association were confirmed, it would not necessarily represent an independent risk factor for binge eating and obesity. This designation would rest on the demonstration that the mutation independently conferred risk for obesity and binge eating—that is, it increased risk for obesity via a mechanism unrelated to binge eating, and vice versa. Similarly, environmental factors—for example, a "toxic" environment with multiple, readily available, highly palatable and calorically dense foods (Brownell, 2002)—may, at least partially independently, promote both binge eating and obesity.

However, although there may be common risk factors, it is increasingly clear that there are risk factors for binge eating that are independent of those for obesity. Bulik and colleagues (2003), in a large population-based twin study using genetic epidemiological methods, found evidence for substantial heritability of both binge eating and obesity, with relatively little overlap of genetic risk factors for the two conditions. More recently, a large-scale study of overweight or obese probands and their first-degree relatives in a community setting found evidence for the existence of BED-specific risk factors that are distinct from other familial risk factors for obesity. Some of these factors may, however, contribute to obesity in individuals with or without full-syndrome BED (Hudson et al., 2006).

In sum, the causal relationships between obesity and BED are complex, and it is likely that no single model of causation accounts for all observed associations. However, it does seem likely that binge eating leads to weight gain over time, whereas the idea that obesity leads to the emergence of binge eating, via dieting, in those who are not otherwise at risk is less clearly supported.

Does the Distinction between Obese BED and Non-BED Matter for Treatment?

The differences between obese subjects with BED and those without BED in psychological and medical comorbidity, past history, and natural course have been reviewed elsewhere in this volume (see Chapter 2). These differences, as well as the possible causal relationships among obesity, dieting, and binge eating, raise questions of great practical importance. Does the treatment response of obese individuals with BED differ from that of non–binge eaters? And should obese individuals with BED who are primarily seeking weight loss receive different treatment than non–binge eaters or additional treatments to address behavioral and psychological components of their disorder?

Do Obese Individuals with BED Respond Differently to Weight Loss Treatment Than Obese Non–Binge Eaters?

Studies of individuals seeking treatment for obesity have provided a relatively clear answer to this question. Recent summaries of the literature (Stunkard & Allison, 2003; Teixeira et al., 2005; Wonderlich et al., 2003) suggest that, with few exceptions, obese individuals with BED do not fare differently than obese individuals without BED in weight loss treatments, either by dropping out more frequently or responding less well, although binge eating may pose a risk for weight regain (Elfhag & Rössner, 2005). There are hints in some weight loss studies that subjects with BED or related conditions may drop out more frequently (LaPorte, 1992; Marcus et al., 1988; Teixeira et al., 2004; Wadden et al., 1992), but this has not been borne out by other obesity treatment studies (de Zwaan et al., 2005b; Gladis et al., 1998b; Ho, 1995). And although one study reported somewhat lower weight loss in binge eaters versus non–binge eaters during CBT–weight control treatment (Marchesini et al., 2002), and at least one study using a liquid VLCD found subjects with BED to be at higher risk for having a poor outcome (Yanovski et al., 1994), most studies did not report differences in mean weight loss between subjects with and without BED (de Zwaan et al., 2005b; Gladis et al., 1998b; LaPorte, 1992; Raymond et al., 2002; Telch & Agras, 1993; Tseng et al., 2004; Wadden et al., 1992). Although most studies using medication for obesity management have not rigorously assessed the differential responses of individuals with and without BED, one early study using fluoxetine combined with behavior modification found that binge eaters did not respond differently (Marcus et al., 1990b). Recent large-scale studies using combined clinical trial data (Sherwood et al., 1999) or managed care samples (Linde et al., 2004) have suggested that BED may be weakly or indirectly associated with poorer weight loss, particularly in obese women. These studies suggested that depression or dysphoria, which is often associated with BED, may be a more powerful predictor. It is important to note that most of the above studies recruited subjects who were primarily interested in weight loss; those with BED were identified during the screening and evaluation process. This may represent a different group of individuals than those who present to eating disorder centers specifically for treatment of binge eating.

The evidence concerning the response of obese binge eaters versus non–binge eaters to surgical treatment for obesity is summarized elsewhere in this volume (see Chapter 6).

Do Obese Individuals with BED Benefit from Specialized Treatments More Than from Standard Weight Control Treatment?

Although there have been many studies of various forms of psychotherapy in patients with BED, most of whom were also overweight or obese (see Chapter 7), fewer studies have specifically compared weight control treatment with specialized eating-disorder-based interventions or have examined the additive effects of these approaches. One important dimension of outcome that could theoretically be augmented by specific attention to binge eating is weight loss. Interestingly, several studies comparing cognitive or nondieting approaches with behavioral weight loss treatment reported no, or minimal, weight loss with either treatment (Goodrick et al., 1998; Grilo & Masheb, 2005; Tanco et al., 1998). Other studies found short and/or long-term weight loss to be greater with behavioral weight loss compared to cognitive treatment (Marcus et al., 1995b; Nauta et al., 2000). A different approach to this question is to combine elements of behavioral weight loss with interventions specific to binge eaters. Porzelius and colleagues (1995) found that patients with severe binge eating had a more favorable weight course with weight loss treatment modified to address binge-eating problems. Devlin and colleagues (2005) found that individual CBT did not yield additional weight loss in subjects with BED who received group behavioral weight loss treatment, although the group treatment had been modified to address binge eating, and weight loss overall was minimal. Using a somewhat different design, Agras and colleagues (1994) found that (1) short-term (3-month) weight loss in subjects with BED was superior in subjects receiving group weight loss treatment compared to group CBT, and (2) subjects receiving 3 months of CBT followed by 6 months of weight loss treatment fared no differently, in weight loss at the end of treatment or at 36-week follow-up, than subjects receiving 9 months of weight loss treatment. Thus, overall, there is very little evidence to suggest that eating-disorder-specific approaches are superior or significantly add to standard weight control approaches when weight loss is the desired outcome. An important consideration in interpreting this literature is that "standard" weight loss treatments increasingly address elements of binge eating, encourage greater flexibility in food selection, promote self-acceptance, and focus on long-term moderate lifestyle changes, which may lessen the contrast between "weight-control-centered" and "eating-disorder-centered" approaches.

A related question is whether cognitive or nondieting approaches, compared to behavioral weight loss treatment, confer tangible benefits with regard to binge eating or psychological symptoms. Here the case for specialized treatments is stronger, with several studies demonstrating superiority for specialized eating-disorder-centered approaches in the short term (Agras et al., 1994; Grilo & Masheb, 2005; Tanco et al., 1998) or long term (Nauta et al., 2000). Devlin and colleagues (2005) found that individual CBT administered in combination with group behavioral weight control treatment adapted for BED conferred greater reduction in binge eating frequency, and this difference was apparent over a 2-year period following CBT (Devlin et al., 2007). In keeping with this finding, a preliminary report from Grilo and colleagues (2006) suggested that group CBT was significantly superior to group behavioral weight loss (BWL) in curbing binge eating, although neither treatment yielded clinically significant weight loss. The sequence of CBT followed by BWL showed little added benefit compared to either CBT or BWL. In contrast to these findings, an earlier study found that binge eating treatment did not reduce binge eating more than weight loss treatment (Porzelius et al., 1995).

A theoretical issue is whether weight loss treatment might, by encouraging increased dietary restraint, promote the onset of binge eating. This outcome has, in fact, been demonstrated *not* to be the case in individuals without a past history of binge eating (Wadden et al., 2004). Whether this is the case in individuals with a past history of BED or related conditions, who are not currently binge eating, is not yet known.

A related final question is whether the presence of binge eating may merit recognition by clinicians, not in the treatment of obesity but in the prevention of obesity. The evidence suggesting that binge eating may promote weight gain and obesity is summarized above. In particular, a recent large-scale epidemiological study suggests that binge eating among adolescents may increase the risk of obesity and eating disorders at 5-year follow-up (Neumark-Sztainer et al., 2006). By extension, therefore, the presence of binge eating would, in fact, matter in those who are not yet, but at risk for, becoming obese.

In sum, the available evidence suggests that, although the distinction between obese BED and obese non-BED may have limited significance in determining suitability for weight loss treatment, there are hints that modifications of treatment or adjunctive treatment for binge eaters may have benefits in ameliorating behavioral and/or psychological symptoms.

Summary

Although a great deal has been learned regarding the relationship between BED and obesity during the past decade, there are aspects of this relationship that remain incompletely understood. Epidemiological studies suggest that a considerable number of normal-weight binge eaters exist, who have many of the clinical features of obese patients with BED and yet often fail to seek treatment. The question of whether binge eating is best regarded as a problem in its own right or as an associated feature of psychological distress in certain vulnerable and, in some cases, obesity-prone individuals has yet to be satisfactorily studied. The causal relationships between obesity and BED are not fully understood. However, there is mounting evidence that unchecked binge eating may be associated with a less favorable weight course. The evidence suggesting that obesity promotes binge eating, mediated in part by dieting, is less clear. There are likely to be genetic factors that increase risk for both obesity and binge eating and may overlap only to a limited extent. Finally, the diagnosis of BED seems to have limited value in clinical decision making when weight reduction is the goal of treatment, but may be important in treatment selection in situations in which the behavioral or psychological features of the syndrome are more prominent. However, the paucity of long-term studies in this area limits confidence with which recommendations can be made regarding whether and how a BED diagnoses should be taken into account in treatment planning.

CHAPTER 4

Eating Behavior, Psychobiology, Medical Risks, and Pharmacotherapy of Binge-Eating Disorder

The purpose of this chapter is to review four interesting and related areas concerning BED. These areas are linked by a focus on a presumed relationship to biological and medical issues, including pharmacotherapy. The first area concerns binge eating behavior per se; this discussion focuses primarily on the feeding laboratory studies that have been done on patients with BED. Such research may point to underlying dysregulation of the biological systems regulating hunger and satiety. Second, we consider several other psychobiological issues, including genetic factors and peptidergic (protein transmitter) regulation of feeding, which have been studied in patients with BED, and we discuss the implications of these findings for our understanding of the disorder. Third, we turn to the medical complications of BED, not all of which appear to be directly attributable to obesity. Last we discuss the limited, although interesting, pharmacotherapy literature regarding BED.

Eating Behavior in BED

As described in the DSM-IV, binge eating is defined identically for patients with BED and those with BN. The criteria include the requirement that the individual eat a large amount of food that is definitely greater than most individuals would eat during a similar period of time and under similar circumstances, in a discreet period of time, accompanied by a sense of loss of control. This criterion was written at a time when the literature available on BED was quite limited. Since then considerable research has accumulated concerning the eating behavior in patients with BED, some of which suggests that binge eating behavior in BED is different from that seen in patients with BN.

Studying eating behavior is highly problematic. We know that most patients are not accurate reporters of their eating behavior, whether or not they have a weight problem, and in general people tend to underestimate the amount that they eat and overestimate the amount that they exercise. Because of these limitations in self-report measures, some of what we know about actual eating behavior in eating disorders, in general, and in BED patients, in particular, comes from feeding laboratory paradigms, which have been utilized at several research clinics. Although there are obvious problems in using a feeding laboratory paradigm, including expectancy effects, the novelty of the environment, and several other factors, these experiments do suggest that we can gain very interesting information about eating behavior using such techniques.

Several different paradigms have been employed. One, which was originally used by Yanovski and colleagues (1992) and subsequently used in a series of experiments at Columbia University, involves asking subjects to binge eat or not to binge eat when presented with an array of foods. The studies employing this paradigm are summarized in Table 4.1.

As can be seen generally, the sample sizes in these studies were relatively small. However, the results are rather striking in suggesting that subjects with BED consistently eat more than subjects without BED both when instructed to binge eat and when simply asked to eat, and the amounts eaten in the binge-eating paradigm certainly seem to involve a large amount of food. Also, although eating more rapidly than usual is included in the criteria set for BED, in the Goldfein and colleagues (1993) study, subjects with BED ate at a slower rate but for a longer period of time. Also of note, the consumption in the Yanovski and colleagues (1992) study was significantly greater than in the Goldfein and colleagues study. However, the mean BMI in the Yanovski and colleagues study was also larger. This relationship between consumption and BMI was studied further in the Guss and colleagues (2002) study, where both less obese and more obese cohorts were studied. The binge-eating meals of the subjects with BED were larger than their normal meals and, among subjects with BED, the more obese subjects ate significantly more than the less obese subjects.

Research has examined other aspects of the of binge-eating phenomena. Telch and Agras (1996a, 1996b), in two separate experiments, examined negative affect and food deprivation as possible precipitants of binge eating. In the first study a negative affective state was induced in

TABLE 4.1. Feeding Laboratory Studies of Binge Eating

Authors (year)	N	BMI	Binge meal caloric intake	Non–binge meal caloric intake
Yanovski et al. (1992)	9 non-BED	38.8 ± 1.4	2,017 ± 267	1,642 ± 64.5
	10 BED	40.1 ± 3.4	2,964 ± 127	2,345 ± 239
Goldfein et al. (1993)	10 non-BED	31.5 ± 5.4	1,115 ± 318	781 ± 423
	10 BED	33.4 ± 5.1	1,515 ± 393	743 ± 245
Guss et al. (2002)	8 non-BED	30.4 ± 0.5	1,109 ± 88.5	1,007 ± 180
	9 BED	31.1 ± 0.5	1,898 ± 190	1,405 ± 215
	6 non-BED	40.4 ± 0.5	1,239 ± 165	1,091 ± 1,08
	12 BED	41.5 ± 0.9	2,388 ± 193	1,539 ± 162

women with ($n = 15$) and without ($n = 15$) BED, following which they were asked to eat from an array of foods. There was not a significant difference in the amount of food consumed following the negative mood induction, although subjects with BED did consume more than subjects without BED. In the second study food deprivation of 1 hour versus 6 hours was used as a stimulus. Both subjects with and without BED consumed more after the longer period of deprivation, but there were no significant differences between the two groups.

Geliebter and colleagues (2001) used a single-item test meal paradigm in which subjects were asked to eat until they felt "extremely full." Geliebter and colleagues found that subjects with BED ($n = 30$) consumed significantly more than subjects without BED ($n = 55$). Anderson and colleagues (2001), in a study with a modest sample size ($n = 8$ in each group), again found that those with BED consumed more calories than those who did not have BED.

Gosnell and colleagues (2001) evaluated the role of the amount of food and the number of foods presented to subjects as possible precipitants of an eating binge. The sample size here again was modest (BED, $n = 5$; non-BED, $n = 5$). Subjects were presented with either one or two favorite binge foods in either two or four times the amount of their usual intake. Subjects with BED consumed more than subjects without BED, although the difference did not reach statistical significance. Increasing the number and amounts of foods increased intake as well.

Another source of information about eating in BED, given the limitations of cross-sectional designs and laboratory studies, has been studies using ecological momentary assessment (EMA) (Stone & Shiffman, 1994). EMA permits the study of behavior in the natural environment. Participants are signaled at times throughout each day to report on eating, external events, and subjective responses such as affective states (see deVries, 1992). Assessments may focus on very recent experiences (e.g., events in the last 5 minutes) or on events that occurred over longer time frames (e.g., in the last 30 minutes; since the previous assessment). This methodology reduces the recall period considerably, from days/weeks to minutes/hours, thereby reducing biases associated with retrospective recall, and it eliminates the need for subjects to summarize the experiences that have occured throughout a day or week (Stone & Shiffman, 1994). EMA strategies have been used to overcome the limitations of cross-sectional studies in stress and coping (Bolger & Zuckerman, 1995), personality traits and negative affect (Bolger, 1990), depression (Stader & Hokanson, 1998), cigarette smoking (Shiffman et al., 1996), chronic pain (Stone et al., 1996), and asthma (Smyth et al., 1999). Such a methodology allows for the identification of antecedent conditions (e.g., interpersonal events), moderating variables (e.g., means of coping), and outcome (e.g., eating, drinking alcohol) much more effectively than using panel designs, in which the interval between measurement is usually quite long (i.e., weeks or months).

Three recent studies have investigated binge-eating behavior using EMA. Greeno and colleagues (2000) conducted a study of binge-eating antecedents in a sample of obese women. Seventy-nine women collected 1 week of data using palmtop computers. All 41 subjects with BED reported one or more episodes of binge eating. However, 25 of 38 subjects without BED reported at least one binge-eating episode as well. Furthermore, binge-eating episodes did not differ in caloric content between those with and without BED (800 vs. 792 calories, respectively). Also, subjects without BED who reported binge eating did so at a rate that well exceeded the minimum frequency required to meet BED criteria. Greeno and colleagues found a different pattern of predictors for the BED group compared to the group without BED regarding antecedents. For subjects with BED, poor mood, low alertness, poor control over eating, craving sweets, being at home, and being alone all predicted an evening binge, and binge eating in the group without BED was predicted by only three of these factors: poor control over eating, craving sweets, and being at home.

Le Grange and colleagues (2001) conducted a study investigating 35 overweight women who each collected an average of 2 weeks of EMA data on a palmtop computer. They found that subjects reported greater levels of negative affect, lower levels of positive affect, and higher restraint scores prior to binge-eating episodes. In comparing antecedents, they found that the subjects with BED had higher stress and desire to binge scores and were less likely to be at work. Le Grange and colleagues found no differences between groups with and without BED in the frequency of binge-eating episodes.

Wegner and colleagues (2002) studied 28 female subjects who reported binge-eating episodes. Participants recorded mood- and setting-related variables as well as binge-eating episodes. Participants' negative mood was elevated on binge-eating days versus non-binge-eating days. Wegner and colleagues did not find that negative mood increased before a binge-eating episode, nor did it decrease after. When examining mood recordings reported immediately after a binge-eating episode, subjects rated their negative moods significantly higher than they recalled before the binge-eating episode.

The relative contribution of psychological versus biological dysregulation to the eating behaviors seen in patients with BED requires further clarification but appears to be a fruitful area of research focus. How to address the problematic eating patterns and behaviors in those with BED is addressed in Part II of this book. We turn now to an examination of factors that are clearly psychobiological.

Psychobiology of BED

There has also been an interest in exploring possible psychobiological abnormalities in patients with BED that might either predispose to, or develop as a consequence of, the disorder. Ghrelin levels have been shown to correlate with food intake in humans and a variety of other species, and appear to peak prior to meal onset. Because of this temporal factor, there has been interest in studying ghrelin in patients with eating disorders. Studies have shown that patients with obesity tend to have lower ghrelin levels, which are interpreted as the body's attempt to adjust to overnutrition. The available studies have shown that ghrelin levels tend to be low in patients with BED, which is probably attributable to their positive energy balance (Monteleone et al., 2005a; Geliebter et al., 2004a).

There has also been an interest in the endogeneous cannabinoid system that is involved in the control of eating. One of the endogenous ligands (i.e., naturally occurring binding substances) for this system, anandamide, has been shown to be involved in the control of eating behavior in humans. Monteleone and colleagues (2005b) examined levels of the endocannabinoid anandamide in 11 women with BED and in 15 healthy-weight controls. Plasma levels were significantly higher in patients with BED, suggesting possible involvement of this transmitter in the mediation of the rewarding aspects of eating behavior in these subjects.

Relative to the genetics of BED, Monteleone and colleagues (2006) examined whether polymorphisms of the promoter region of the 5HTT serotonin transporter might contribute to a vulnerability to BED, finding that both the L genotype and the LL genotype of the 5HTTPR were significantly more frequent in binge-eating subjects. These results await replication.

An early report by Branson and colleagues (2003) linking binge eating to mutations of the melanocortin-4 receptor (MC4R) system has been challenged because most of the mutations described were inactive (Farooqui et al., 2003) and further studies reported that binge eating is not characteristic of patients with MC4R variants (Hebebrand et al., 2004; Herpertz et al., 2003). Tortorella and colleagues (2005) reported that a large sample of patients with BED, diagnosed according to DSM-IV criteria and who were not selected for obesity did not show evidence of an increased rate of mutations in either the MC4R or the pro-opiomelanocortin gene.

Medical Complications of BED

We turn now to the medical complications of BED, which unfortunately have received very limited attention from researchers. This is somewhat surprising, when one considers two points. First, the myriad medical complications of the purging behavior and severe restrictive eating (as seen in patients with BN and AN) have been described in considerable detail (Mitchell & Crow, 2006). Second, the medical complications of obesity are similarly well described and have received a great deal of emphasis in recent years with the growing prevalence of obesity and obesity-related medical problems (Field et al., 2001).

From the standpoint of medical complications, the central feature of BED in many clinical populations relates to elevated BMI. If increased BMI were the only medical matter of importance, then the medical complications of BED would essentially be those of obesity. However, this is far from clear. Thus, the critical question becomes: Does having BED confer risk for medical problems or impact the severity of medical problems above and beyond the risk conferred by an individual's elevated BMI?

In this section we review general health status, quality of life, and health care utilization as reported by individuals with BED. Then we examine whether BED increases the risk for specific medical illnesses, influences the course of medical illnesses, and whether its treatment improves physical health.

Health Status, Quality of Life, and Health Care Utilization

A small but growing body of evidence in this area suggests that BED in individuals who are obese is associated with diminished health status when compared to individuals who are similarly obese but do not have BED. Johnson and colleagues (2001) screened a large primary care clinic population and found that BED was relatively common, and that the presence of BED was associated with more overall health complaints. Bulik and colleagues (2002) surveyed 2,163 female twins in the Virginia Twin Registry, finding BED in 2.7%. Those with BED had an overall greater level of health dissatisfaction than non-BED controls. Another study of twins, examining both male and female twins, found that overall levels of health impairment were greater in males with BED (but not females), even after controlling for severity of obesity.

A limited amount of work has examined quality of life in BED. Crow and colleagues (2001) compared quality of life in individuals with Type II diabetes with and without BED and found diminished quality of life in the subjects with BED compared to the controls. Specifically, most subscales of the Impact of Weight on Quality of Life Scale (IWQOL; Kolotkin, Head, &

Brookhart, 1997) showed greater impairment in BED. Reiger, Wilfley, Stein, Marino & Crow (2005) examined quality-of-life ratings in a large number of individuals presenting for treatment in a pharmacotherapy study of BED and found greater quality-of-life impairment in those with BED, based on total and subscale scores using a shortened version of the IWQOL (Kolotkin et al., 2001). de Zwaan and colleagues (2002) also reported lower levels of quality of life in subjects with BED, using a sample of participants seeking bariatric surgery.

Recently, Striegel-Moore and colleagues (2005) compared health care utilization in those with BN or BED and those without. These authors reported on a sample of 1,582 women drawn from the community-based National Heart, Lung and Blood Institute Growth and Health Study (1992). The sample was divided into those with no psychiatric disorder ($n = $ 1,072), those with BN or BED ($n = 67$), and those with a non-eating-related psychiatric disorder ($n = 443$). Health care utilization was higher in both the eating disorder and non-eating-disorder psychiatric groups than in the group with no disorder. These two groups of eating- and non-eating-related psychiatric disorders did not differ significantly between them in terms of health care utilization.

BED and the Risk for Specific Medical Problems

It is reasonable to hypothesize that BED carries an increased risk of specific medical problems for several reasons. First, as noted above, a host of medical problems is linked to disordered eating behaviors in AN and BN. Second, there is mounting evidence that the presence of a mood disorder such as major depression carries an elevated risk of specific medical illnesses, including, for example, hypertension (Jonas et al., 1997) and heart disease (Frasure-Smth et al., 1993). Given the elevated rates of comorbid major depression in patients with BED, these patients might face similar risks. In a similar vein, some authors have hypothesized that BED should best be thought of as representing mood or affective symptoms. If this were a valid approach, it too might provide a mechanism by which BED could increase the risk for specific medical problems. Finally, the large eating binges commonly reported by individuals with BED could carry specific risks for some medical problems, including gastrointestinal problems and, conceivably, endocrine/metabolic disturbances.

However, Bulik and colleagues (2002) in their sample of female twins, found that rates of specific medical problems were not elevated compared to controls. On the other hand, Reichborn-Kjennerud and colleagues (2004) found elevated rates of neck/shoulder pain, muscle pain, and low back pain, plus higher rates of pain medicine usage in males with BED compared to males without BED. No studies to date have identified elevated rates of hypertension or heart disease. Thus, this line of thinking is somewhat speculative.

BED and Type II Diabetes Mellitus

An area of particularly active interest has been the possibility of a link between BED and the risk for Type II diabetes mellitus. An early study found relatively high rates of individuals with elevated BES scores (Gormally et al., 1982) in a clinical range (21% of female participants, 9% male participants). Subsequently, Kenardy and colleagues (1994) reported a rate of BED diagnosis of 6% in Type II diabetes subjects.

Following these two initial rating scale-based reports, Crow and colleagues (2001) completed a study using a structured interview, specifically, the Structured Clinical Interview for

DSM-IV (SCID; First et al., 1995). In this study, 25.6% of clinic patients with diabetes met criteria for BED. More recently, Mannucci (2002) reported on a larger sample (156 subjects) assessed using the EDE. In this sample, the rate of BED was only 2.5% in female participants and 0.5% in male participants. However, Herpertz and colleagues (2000) also reported elevated rates of BED in individuals with Type II diabetes mellitus. Similarly, Papelbaum and colleagues (2005), using the SCID in 70 individuals with Type II diabetes mellitus, found a rate of BED of 10%. Most recently, Allison and colleagues (2007) reported on a sample of over 800 participants in the Look Ahead trial, a treatment study for patients with Type II diabetes mellitus. In this large sample using the EDE-Q (the questionnaire version), 5.6% of individuals screened positive, but subsequent confirmatory interviews using the EDE led to only 1.4% of individuals receiving a BED diagnosis (underscoring the problem with questionnaire self-reports as the sole ascertainment tool).

BED and the Course of Medical Illness

The question of how BED affects the course of medical illness again demonstrates the relatively large gaps in the current existing literature. We know that depression increases the likelihood of new-onset heart disease and also adversely impacts the outcome of heart disease (Frasure-Smith et al., 1993). Similarly one might question whether BED has a similar effect. An interesting recent report found altered cardiac parasympathetic function in individuals with BED (Friederich et al., 2005). Although these data do not directly implicate BED in terms of risk for heart disease, they raise important questions for further study.

The influence of other eating disorders such as BN on the course of Type I diabetes mellitus has been well studied, and a limited body of evidence has examined the same question regarding BED in Type II diabetes mellitus. Specifically, one study found evidence of worsened glycemic control in association with BED or disordered eating (Mannucci et al., 2002), but two others have not (Crow et al., 2001; Herpertz et al., 2000).

Successful Treatment of BED and the Course of Medical Illness

One approach to answering the question of how the successful treatment of BED impacts the course of medical illness is to examine the impact of the BED treatment on subsequent glycemic control. This question has been examined in one study that compared group CBT with group nonprescriptive therapy (Kenardy et al., 2002). In both treatment conditions, improvement over the course of treatment was associated with improved glycemic control.

There is also some evidence that treating BED may have a broader impact on health-related quality of life. Marchesini and colleagues (2002) examined the impact of CBT on patients with and without BED and found HRQOL ratings improved following treatment, with greater improvement in those with greater improvement in BED.

Pharmacotherapy for BED

Last, we turn to the pharmacotherapy of BED. Medication treatments represent a potentially useful adjunctive approach for BED. There are a number of reasons why such treatments are appealing (perhaps, in some ways, more appealing than psychotherapy). First, it is probably easier to train providers to effectively prescribe psychotropic medications for BED than it is to train providers in empirically supported psychotherapies for BED. The medications that have been studied for BED treatment are frequently prescribed by nonpsychiatric physicians for a variety of other indications. By contrast, there is evidence to suggest that therapies that were carefully tested for BN and BED are used relatively rarely by therapists (Crow et al., 1999), and therapists frequently are not carefully trained in them (Mussell et al., 2000). Additionally, at least in theory, medications might provide specific efficacy for two types of comorbidity frequently seen with BED: psychiatric comorbidity and obesity.

The work examining pharmacotherapy for BED has grown out of two other bodies of literature (and, perhaps, from two separate conceptualizations of BED): studies of BN, and studies of obesity. One line of research has focused on those medications previously shown to provide benefit for binge eating as it occurs in BN, presumably via impact on affect or anxiety, or perhaps on impulsivity or obsessionality. The second line of research has examined those medications used for obesity, usually as appetite suppressants.

In providing clinical BED treatment, at least two desired clinical outcomes must be kept in mind: weight loss and cessation of binge eating. In fact, evidence suggests that the goal of weight loss may be more important than the goal of binge-eating cessation for many individuals seeking treatment (Brody et al., 2005)

In this section we review medications studied in blinded, placebo-controlled trials. The results of these studies are summarized in Table 4.2, and the studies are discussed individually: first the antidepressant agents, then appetite suppressant and other weight loss drugs.

Antidepressants

Tricyclic Antidepressants

Three studies have examined the role of tricyclic antidepressants in the treatment of BED. The first of these examined desipramine (McCann & Agras, 1990). In this 12-week study, 30 subjects were randomized to desipramine or placebo. Desipramine performed significantly better than placebo, resulting in a 63% decrease in binge-eating frequency (vs. a 16% increase with placebo) and 60% abstinence rate at end of treatment (vs. 15% for placebo). Both treatment groups lost some weight, with the amount of weight loss being greater in the desipramine group than with placebo (3.5 kg vs. 1.2 kg). Alger and colleagues (1991) compared imipramine to placebo (as well as naltrexone, in another arm of the same study) over an 8-week period. A modest degree of weight loss was seen in the imipramine group (0.6%) in subjects receiving up to 200 mg per day. By contrast, a 1.4% increase in weight was seen in the placebo group. Finally, Laederach-Hoffman and colleagues (1999) also examined imipramine in another 8-week trial, dosing the drug at 75 mg per day. A 73% decrease in binge-eating frequency was seen in the active treatment group, versus 28% with placebo. Similarly, the imipramine group lost 2.2 kg, whereas the placebo group gained a very small amount of weight.

Selective Serotonin Reuptake Inhibitors

A larger body of work has examined the use of selective serotonin reuptake inhibitors (SSRIs) in BED, and most of the marketed SSRIs have been studied. The first study to examine these agents focused on fluoxetine (Marcus et al., 1990b). In this 52-week study employing a dose of

TABLE 4.2. Blinded, Placebo-Controlled Pharmacotherapy Trials in BED

Authors (year)	Drug	N	Duration	Dose	% abstinent	% decrease in binge eating	Weight loss (% or kg)
McCann & Agras (1990)	Desipramine	30	12 wk	25–300mg	60% (vs. 15%)	63% (vs. 16% ↑)	3.5 kg (vs. 1.2 kg)
Marcus et al. (1990b)[a]	Fluoxetine	45	52 wk	60 mg	NR	NR	13.9 kg (vs. 0.6 kg ↑)
Stunkard et al. (1996a)	d-Fenfluramine	28	8 wk	15–30 mg	NR	73% (vs. 0.0%)	None in either group
Hudson (1998)	Fluvoxamine	85	9 wk	50–300 mg	45% (vs. 24%)	NR	1.3 kg (vs. 0.4 kg)
Alger et al. (1991)	Imipramine or naltrexone	33	8 wk	50–200 (Imi) 50–100 (Nltrx)	NR	NR	0.6% Imi 0.6% Nltrx (vs. 1.4 ↑)
Laederach-Hoffman et al. (1999)	Imipramine	31	8 wk	75 mg	NR	73% (vs. 28%)	2.2 kg (vs. 0.2 kg ↑)
McElroy et al. (2000)	Sertraline	34	6 wk	50–100mg	54% (vs. 15%)	85% (vs. 45%)	5.6 kg (vs. 2.4 kg)
Arnold et al. (2002)	Fluoxetine	60	6 wk	20–80 mg	45%	70% (vs. 56%)	3.3 kg (vs. 0.7 kg)
McElroy et al. (2003a)	Topiramate	61	14 wk	50–600 mg	64% (vs. 30%)	94% (vs. 46%)	5.9 (vs. 1.2 kg ↑)
McElroy et al. (2003b)	Citalopram	38	6 wk	20–60 mg	47% (vs. 21%)	67% (vs. 40%)	2.1 kg (0.2 kg ↑)
Pearlstein et al. (2003)	Fluvoxamine	20	12 wk	Up to 300 mg			
Appolinario et al. (2003)	Sibutramine	60	12 wk	15 mg	52% (vs. 32%)	66% (vs. 41%)	7.4 kg (vs. 1.4 kg ↑)
Golay et al. (2005)	Orlistat	89	24 wk	360 mg	82% (vs. 73%)	NR	7.4% (vs. 2.3%)
Wilfley et al. (2006)	Sibutramine	304	24 wk	10–15 mg	NR	85% (vs. 77%)	4.3 kg (vs. 0.8 kg)
McElroy et al. (2007)	Topiramate	407	16 wk	25–400 mg	58% (vs. 29%)	72% (vs. 47%)	BMI ↓ 1.6 kg/m^2 (vs. 0.08 ↓)
Milano et al. (2005)	Sibutramine	20	12 wk	10 mg	NR	77% (vs. 6%)	4.5 kg (vs. 0.6 kg)

Note. For % abstinent, % decrease in binge eating, and % weight loss, placebo figures are listed in parentheses. NR, not reported.
[a] Marcus et al. (1990b) included 22 binge eaters + 23 non–binge-eating obese subjects.

60 mg per day, a clinically and statistically significant weight loss was seen (13.9 kg) as compared to the placebo group, which experienced a 0.6 kg weight gain. Subsequently, Hudson and colleagues (1998) examined fluvoxamine in a somewhat larger trial (85 subjects) receiving 9 weeks of treatment. Fluvoxamine was dosed at up to 300 mg per day. Forty-five percent of fluvoxamine-treated subjects achieved abstinence from binge eating versus 24% for the placebo group. A modest weight loss was seen (1.3 kg vs. 0.4 kg for placebo). Fluvoxamine was again examined in another small study (20 subjects; Pearlstein et al., 2003). In this 12-week study, the majority of subjects in both the active treatment group and the placebo group became abstinent, but statistical differences between active treatment and placebo were not seen. McElroy and colleagues (2000) examined sertraline in a dose of 50–100 mg per day given over a 6-week period. Higher abstinence rates were seen in the active treatment patients (54% vs. 15% for placebo) as well as greater overall diminishment in binge-eating frequency (85% for sertraline vs. 45% for placebo). In addition, an impressive weight loss was seen (5.6 kg vs. 2.4 kg for placebo). Fluoxetine was again studied by Arnold and colleagues (2002), who randomized 60 subjects to a 6-week period of treatment with fluoxetine, up to 80 mg per day. Forty-five percent of fluoxetine-treated patients achieved abstinence from binge eating, and fluoxetine treatment was associated with a 3.3 kg weight loss (vs. 0.7 kg for placebo). Citalopram was investigated by McElroy and colleagues (2003b). This 6-week trial examined doses up to 60 mg per day and demonstrated abstinence in 47% of citalopram-treated patients. In addition, citalopram-treated patients experienced a 2.1 kg weight loss (vs. 0.2 kg weight gain with placebo).

Weight Loss Agents

The first study of a weight loss agent for BED examined the utility of *d*-fenfluramine (Stunkard et al., 1996a). This paper is now of historical interest, given that *d*-fenfluramine is no longer marketed due to concerns about the drug causing valvular heart disease. However, the study is also of considerable theoretical interest because of the results. Binge eating decreased by 73% in the active drug group; binge eating did not change in the placebo group. However, on average, weight was unchanged at the end of 8 weeks of treatment in both active drug and placebo conditions. This was quite a surprising finding, as one might well have imagined that marked changes in binge-eating frequency would be associated with some change in weight, especially in light of the demonstrated efficacy of *d*-fenfluramine in obesity treatment.

Subsequent to that trial, more recently developed and marketed weight loss agents have also received increasing attention. In particular, three trials of sibutramine have now been reported. In the first report, 60 subjects received either sibutramine (15 mg/day) or placebo for 12 weeks (Appolinario et al., 2003). Fifty-two percent of subjects on sibutramine achieved abstinence from binge eating, versus 32% with placebo; this difference was statistically significant. Significant weight loss was also seen in the drug-treated group (7.4 kg vs. 1.4 kg with placebo). Milano and colleagues (2005) subsequently reported on a sample of 20 subjects randomized to placebo or sibutramine, again for a 12-week period, but this time at a dose of 10 mg per day. A 77% decrease in binge eating was observed (vs. 6% with placebo), and again a substantial weight loss occurred (4.5 kg vs. 0.6 kg with placebo). Finally, Wilfley and Crow (2006) have reported on a longer multicenter trial of sibutramine. This study randomized 304 subjects to 24 weeks of treatment with a dose of 10–15 mg of sibutramine per day. An 85%

decrease in binge eating was reported versus 77% for placebo, and a modest weight loss was seen (4.3 kg vs. 0.8 kg for placebo). In each of these trials, modest elevations in blood pressure and pulse were seen, in keeping with those typically encountered with sibutramine treatment, but in other respects the agent was fairly well tolerated.

Three studies have now examined the use of topiramate for BED. Topiramate is used primarily as an anticonvulsant, but it was noted to be associated with weight loss in epilepsy trials, and has thus received attention as a potential agent both for obesity treatment and for the treatment of BED. McElroy and colleagues (2003a) initially reported on a study of 61 individuals with BED. These participants received 14 weeks of treatment with topiramate or placebo, ranging from 50 to 600 mg per day. Sixty-four percent of subjects became abstinent on topiramate versus 30% on placebo. Marked decreases in overall rates of binge eating also were reported, with a 94% decrease in those receiving the active drug versus 46% for placebo. In addition, a 5.9 kg weight loss was experienced by topiramate-treated patients, versus a 1.2 kg weight gain after 14 weeks in those receiving placebo. McElroy and colleagues (2004) subsequently reported on the 1-year outcome of participants in their topiramate study who received open-label drug treatment. Individuals who received the active drug during the initial 14 weeks of the study generally maintained the improvements in binge eating they had experienced during the trial and also maintained the same general degree of weight loss they had already achieved, with little evidence of decay of that weight loss over the follow-up year. Those who had received placebo initially were randomized to active drug, and they achieved similar benefits to those observed in the initial double-blind phase with the topiramate-treated group. These data are relatively unique and quite useful, but it should be noted that the sample size was modest in this study.

Subsequently, McElroy and colleagues (2007) reported on a much larger trial with 407 participants, who received 16 weeks of treatment with topiramate, up to 400 mg per day, or placebo. Abstinence rates were significantly greater in the active-drug-treated group (58% vs. 29% for placebo), as were decreases in overall binge eating (72% vs. 47%). A 1.6 kg/m^2 decrease in BMI was observed with the active drug (compared to a decrease of only 0.08 kg/m^2 for placebo). In addition, topiramate was studied in combination with CBT in a placebo-controlled 21-week trial (Claudino et al., 2006). Topiramate plus CBT was associated with greater weight loss (6.8 kg vs. 0.9 kg) and higher abstinence rates (84% vs. 61%) than placebo plus CBT.

One report discussed the use of orlistat for BED (Golay et al., 2005). In this 24-week study subjects received up to 360 mg per day of orlistat. Similar rates of abstinence from binge eating were observed at the end of treatment (82% with active drug, 73% with placebo) but greater weight loss was seen in association with orlistat treatment (7.4% vs. 2.3% for placebo).

Treatment Approach

How does one translate this literature into a cohesive treatment approach? When should pharmacological treatments be used, and which drugs should be used? Should pharmacological treatments be initiated at the time that psychotherapy or behavioral weight loss begins, or should they be based only on treatment response (or lack thereof). If so, are decisions to be made based on degree of weight loss, comorbid psychiatric symptoms, degree of changes in binge eating or target eating-disordered cognitions? Finally, what is the appropriate duration of treatment? These issues are addressed below.

When Should Treatment Be Initiated Relative to Psychotherapy or Behavioral Weight Loss?

First, it is worth stressing that the answer to this question is somewhat unclear. The impact of pharmacological agents added to psychotherapies has been variable in the psychiatric literature. These studies are summarized in Table 4.3. In the treatment of BED, two studies published thus far do not suggest any benefit from adding fluoxetine to CBT (Devlin et al., 2005; Grilo et al., 2005b). In these studies, medication and psychotherapy were initiated simultaneously, so questions about treating psychotherapy nonresponders were not addressed. A third study, in which orlistat or placebo was added to CBT, did find greater weight loss with active drug and greater end-of-treatment (but not 3-month follow-up) abstinence from binge eating (Grilo et al., 2005a).

Decisions about treatment sequencing hinge, in part, on treatment goals. If substantial weight loss is a goal, weight loss drugs might be considered early in treatment. One can expect minimal benefit in terms of weight loss for most psychotherapy-treated patients, based on the existing literature. Furthermore, significant weight loss in response to pharmacological treatment has been seen only with a limited number of agents (e.g., orlistat, topiramate, sibutramine). Several other agents, primarily antidepressants, have shown substantial improvement in binge eating without significant changes in weight loss. On the other hand, those agents may be helpful for comorbid psychiatric problems that would be unaffected by weight loss agents.

In considering the role of medication treatment, it may also be worth considering which specific psychotherapeutic treatments are available for a given patient. Empirically studied treatments such as CBT have not been widely disseminated and are often not available. It may be reasonable to institute pharmacotherapy in place of untested and unproven psychotherapeutic approaches.

What Constitutes an Adequate Trial of Pharmacotherapy for BED?

Again, the answer to this question is really unknown. Experience of practitioners in this field often assumes that adequate treatment for BED is unlikely to involve a substantially *shorter* period of time than is seen for an uncomplicated episode of depression (i.e., close to a year or perhaps more). Thus, 12 months of treatment is a commonly sought goal. This goal, however, is most appropriate if the main focus of treatment is cessation of binge eating. In the treatment of obesity, it is clear that prolonged response to pharmacological treatment requires prolonged pharmacotherapy. There is no particular reason to believe that this would be any different in the presence of binge eating. Thus, if weight loss is a prominent goal (and if weight loss is achieved with medication), strong consideration should be given to long-term pharmacotherapy to help maintain such weight loss.

Summary

Subjects with BED have been studied using feeding laboratory paradigms and EMA. These individuals clearly eat more than obese model controls, and there is some evidence that negative affective stress may precipitate binge-eating episodes. A report linking BED to mutations of the MC4R receptor have not been replicated.

TABLE 4.3. Combination Studies of CBT Plus Medication

Authors (year)	Drug	N	Duration	Dose	% abstinent	% decrease in binge eating	Weight loss (kg)
Devlin et al. (2005)	Fluoxetine	116	20 wk	60 mg	62% (CBT) 33% (no CBT)	85% (Flx + CBT) 78% (Plc + CBT) 70% (Flx) 61% (Plc)	4.1 kg 1.9 kg 1.9 kg 2.4 kg
Grilo et al. (2005a)	Orlistat	50	12 wk	360 mg	64% 36% (Plc + CBT GSH)	79.1% (vs. 71.9% Plc/CBT GSH)	3.5 kg (vs. 1.5 kg Plc + CBT GSH)
Grilo et al. (2005b)	Fluoxetine	108	16 wk	60 mg	29% (Flx) 55% (Flx/CBT) 30% (Plc) 73% (Plc/CBT)	43% (Flx) 69% (Flx/CBT) 46% (Plc) 89% (Plc/CBT)	–.8 kg/m² (Flx) .8 kg/m² (Flx/CBT) 0 (Plc) .8 kg/m² (Plc/CBT)
Claudino et al. (2006)	Topirimate	73	21 wk	200 mg	84% (vs. 61% Plc/CBT)	NR	6.8 kg (vs. 0.9 kg (Plc/CBT)

Note. Flx, fluoxetine; Plc, placebo; CBT, cognitive-behavioral therapy; GSH, guided self-help; NR, not reported.

BED appears to adversely impact health status and may be associated with increased health care utilization. Conflicting results have suggested mild to marked increases in the risk for Type II diabetes mellitus in those with BED. Perhaps surprisingly, there is little evidence to link binge eating with worsened glycemic control. It remains to be clarified whether successful treatment of BED will impact health status, and if so, whether such impact is independent of benefits from weight loss.

There is ample support for the use of antidepressants and weight loss agents to diminish binge eating in BED. However, weight loss has often been modest, especially with antidepressants. Evidence regarding the added benefit from medication for eating disorder target symptoms, over and above that seen with CBT, has been inconsistent. Still, medications are a useful part of the BED treatment armamentarium, especially when empirically validated therapies are unavailable or psychiatric comorbidity is prominent.

CHAPTER 5

Binge-Eating Disorder and Bariatric Surgery

The topic of BED has refocused interest on the relationship between eating pathology and obesity. There has also been a growing awareness that many patients who are candidates for bariatric surgery also suffer from problems with binge eating and may meet full criteria for BED. This reality raises questions as to whether or not comorbid BED might pose certain additional risks and might compromise long-term outcome of the surgery.

In this chapter we first provide an overview of the bariatric surgery procedures commonly practiced, for those who might be less knowledgeable about this area. We then discuss data on BED patients being assessed for bariatric surgery and discuss the implications of comorbid BED for surgery outcome both in the short and long term.

Bariatric Surgery Procedures

As has been widely recognized, the prevalence of obesity has been markedly escalating in the United States and in many parts of the world (Ogden et al., 2003). This escalation is particularly true of patients with a BMI greater than 40 kg/m², who can be considered the extremely obese and who are at a markedly increased risk for obesity-related medical complications (Bray, 2003). Such risks include hypertension, dyslipidemia, increased intra-abdominal pressure resulting in urinary incontinence and gastroesophageal reflux, sleep apnea, various hormonal abnormalities (including amenorrhea and problems conceiving), osteoarthritis, several types of malignancies (including cancers of the colon, uterus, and breast), as well as a markedly increased risk of developing Type II diabetes mellitus (Bray, 2003; Maggio & Pi-Sunyer, 2003). Given the rising prevalence of obesity, the growing awareness of its untoward health consequences, and the finding that many of the traditional psychosocial and pharmacological interventions for obesity seem to have a marginal impact on long-term body weight, the use of bariatric surgery procedures has grown dramatically over the last few years and is like to continue to expand (Latifiet al., 2002).

As with most medical and surgical interventions, the forms of bariatric surgery employed have been modified substantially over the last 40 years. The first procedure to be widely utilized was the jejunoileal bypass (JIB; see Figure 5.1), which resulted in profound malabsorption and was frequently associated with a number of severe medical complications, including protein calorie malnutrition, various vitamin and mineral deficiencies, hypocalcemia with bone loss, bone pain, and diarrhea (Balsinger et al., 2000). Although this procedure resulted in substantial weight loss, the side effects were unacceptable, and it has now been abandoned as a preferred approach.

Shortly after World War II a variety of purely restrictive (limiting gastric capacity) procedures were introduced, including the horizontal gastroplasty (see Figure 5.2), and later the vertical-banded gastroplasty (see Figure 5.3), wherein the gastric outlet was reinforced with a mesh collar to prevent enlargement of the stoma. The advantage to these procedures was that they resulted in essentially no metabolic complications, but the intake of high-calorie foods in patients who had undergone such procedures was essentially unlimited, particularly in the form of sweet drinks, and many times this resulted in insufficient weight loss. In 1969 Mason and Ito introduced the gastric bypass, which included elements of both malabsorption and gastric restriction (see Figure 5.4).

This surgery was later modified to include a roux-en-Y configuration and complete staple-line transection to avoid eventual staple line failure (see Figure 5.5).

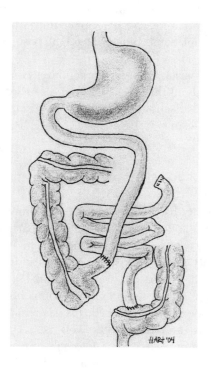

FIGURE 5.1. Jejunoileal bypass.

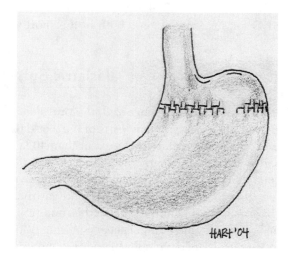

FIGURE 5.2. Horizontal gastroplasty.

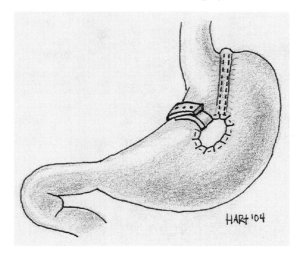

FIGURE 5.3. Vertical-banded gastroplasty.

The roux-en-Y gastric bypass is now the most commonly performed bariatric surgery procedure in the United States. Weight loss with this procedure is substantial: generally, a loss of 60–80% of excess weight with some regain after 18–24 months. Short-term complications include bleeding and the development of blood clots as well as leaking at the anastamotic site; long-term complications include anemia, B_{12}, iron, and calcium deficiencies, as well as dumping syndrome (wherein patients feel faint and may experience diarrhea). Roux-en-Y bypasses are now commonly performed laproscopically (Courcoulas et al., 2003).

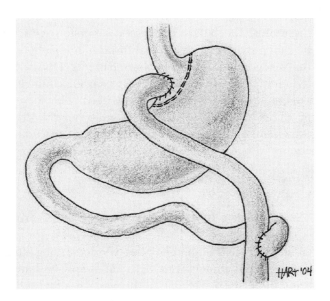

FIGURE 5.4. Gastric bypass.

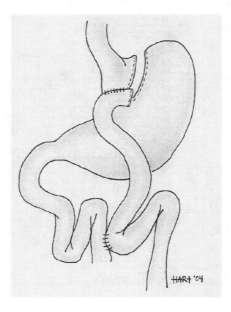

FIGURE 5.5. Roux-en-Y gastric bypass.

Most recently, gastric banding techniques have been introduced to provide a restrictive approach that does not induce malabsorption. These gastric banding procedures are performed laproscopically and have become particularly popular worldwide and are now gaining acceptance in the United States (Steffen et al., 2003). Weight loss with this procedure is more limited than with bypass, but the procedure is fairly easy to reverse and technically not difficult to complete (see Figure 5.6).

For "super-obese" patients, the biliary pancreatic diversion with duodenal switch has been introduced, which again provides marked malabsorption but has a high complication rate, and is reserved for the most severely ill, severely obese patients. Disadvantages include ulcerations, anemia, mineral/vitamin deficiencies, and protein calorie malnutrition (see Figure 5.7).

Many of the medical comorbidities that accompany obesity have been shown to improve and at times to normalize after bariatric surgery, often quite rapidly. Because of this success, obesity experts are turning increasingly toward bariatric surgery procedures as a treatment for their severely obese patients who are unable to lose weight or maintain weight loss by other, more traditional means.

Psychosocial Assessment in Bariatric Surgery Patients with BED

Health-related quality of life is a construct that has received increasing attention in the medical literature, allowing researchers and clinicians to focus not simply on longevity but the quality of life of individuals during their lifespan. Some of this work has focused on bariatric surgical procedures. Research has shown that compared to individuals in the general population, surprisingly bariatric surgery candidates report many more difficulties in various areas of health-related quality of life, including emotional functioning, bodily pain, and general overall health

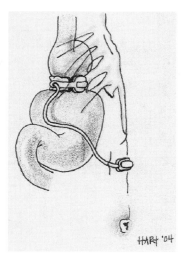

FIGURE 5.6. Gastric banding.

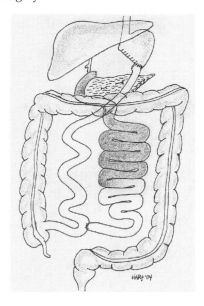

FIGURE 5.7. Biliary pancreatic diversion with duodenal switch.

(de Zwaan et al., 2003b). Among obese individuals seeking bariatric surgery, health-related quality of life appears to vary significantly depending on the presence or absence of BED. Those with BED show significantly more impairment in both physical and mental functioning (de Zwaan et al., 2003b).

Another issue concerns the ability of obese individuals with BED to lose weight in traditional weight loss programs. It is generally accepted that patients with BED, compared to BMI-matched controls, tend to have an earlier onset of obesity, an unstable weight history, and generally higher rates of psychopathology (Marcus et al., 1990a; Spitzer et al., 1993b; Yanovski et al., 1993). However, patients with BED do not typically have more difficulty losing weight in traditional weight loss programs in most reported research (Gormally et al., 1982; Ho et al., 1995; Keefe et al., 1984), although there is some evidence that these individuals are more likely to drop out of weight loss treatment and are more likely to regain weight after treatment (Marcus et al., 1988).

Binge-Eating Behavior before and after Bariatric Surgery

Various authors have examined the prevalence of binge eating and full BED in individuals prior to bariatric surgery, using a variety of self-report and clinician-administered instruments. These data are summarized in Table 5.1. As can be seen, depending on the nature of the data collected and the method of collecting it, markedly disparate rates of binge eating and BED have been ascertained in patients who are candidates for bariatric surgery, making it difficult to come up with a firm prevalence figure. However, overall, one must conclude that BED does appear to be a substantial problem in many patients who undergo bariatric surgery.

TABLE 5.1. Binge Eating/BED before and after Bariatric Surgery

Authors (year)	Site	Procedures	N	Baseline BE	Baseline BED	Follow-up BE	Follow-up BED	Duration
Adami et al. (1995)	Genoa	"Bariatric surgery"	92	69%	47%	—	—	—
Busetto et al. (1996)	Padova	Lap band	80	—	13%	—	—	—
Adami et al. (1996)	Genoa	BPD	65	64%	—	9%	—	2 yr
Hsu et al. (1996)	Pitt	VBG	24	—	38%	—	21%	3.5 yr
Hsu et al. (1997)	Tufts	VBG	27	—	48%	—	7%	21 mo
Kalarchian et al. (1999)	Rutgers	RYGBP	64	39%	—	—	—	—
Saunders et al. (2004)	Virginia	RYGBP	125	61%	—	—	—	—
Powers et al. (1999)	University of South Florida	"Gastric restriction"	116	52%	16%	0%	—	5.5 yr
Kalarchian et al. (1999)	University of Pittsburgh	RYGBP	50	44%	—	0%	—	4 mo
Lang et al. (2002)	Zürich	Lap band	66	64%	11%	71%	—	12 mo
Burgmer et al. (2005)	Essen	Lap band	149	20%[a]	2%	—	—	—
Wadden et al. (2001)	University of Pennsylvania	RYGBP	115	10%	27%	—	—	—
Dymek et al. (2001)	University of Chicago	RYGBP	32	—	32%	—	0%	6 mo
Mitchell et al. (2001)	Neuropsychiatric Research Institute	RYGBP	78	197	49%	—	7%	14 yr
Busetto et al. (2005)	Padova	Lap band	260	—	29%	—	—	3 yr
Kalarchian et al. (2002)	University of Pittsburgh	RYGBP	99	—	—	46%	—	2–7 yr
Hsu et al. (2002)	Tufts	VBG	37	25%	11%	—	—	—
Delgado et al. (2002)	Pontevedra (Spain)	RYGBP	80	—	17%	—	—	—
Sanchez-Johnsen et al. (2003)	University of Chicago		210	—	26%	—	—	—
de Zwaan et al. (2003b)	Neuropsychiatric Research Institute	RYGBP	110	39%	17%	—	—	—
Boan et al. (2004)	Duke	RYGBP	40	30%	—	0%	—	6 mo
Green et al. (2004)	University of Chicago	RYGBP	65	50%	26%	—	—	—
Malone & Alger-Mayer (2004)	State University of New York	RYGBP	109	52%		55%		12 mo
Larsen et al. (2004)	Utrecht	Lap band	93/160	56%	—	37%	—	—
Mazzeo et al. (2005)	Virginia Commonwealth University	RYGBP	388	—	35%	—	—	—
Allison et al. (2006)	University of Pennsylvania	—	215	—	4%	—	—	—

Note. BE, binge eating; BED, binge-eating disorder; BPD, bilropancreatic diversion; VBG, vertical-banded gastroplasty; RYGBP, roux-en-Y gastric bypass; lap band, laproscopic banding.
[a]Including grazing.

One of the major problems in assessing eating behavior, in general, and patients' status postbariatric surgery procedures, in particular, is defining what actually constitutes "normal" versus "abnormal" eating behavior. We know that patients who undergo bariatric surgery procedures, particularly those undergoing such procedures as roux-en-Y gastric bypass, will have marked changes in their eating behavior and will require the frequent intake of small amounts of food, with extensive chewing before swallowing. However, what actually constitutes "normal"? One predominant eating behavior is binge eating. As noted, the frequency of binge eating and full BED varies widely among sample of individuals seeking bariatric surgery (de Zwaan, 2001), with a range from a low 1% to a high of 49%. There is some suggestion in this literature that the most current studies report somewhat lower levels, probably owing to more careful methodology and better definitions of this behavior. However, it must be remembered that many patients minimize their eating problems prior to surgery because they want to be approved for the procedure (Glinski et al., 2001).

Another behavior that needs to be discussed is "grazing," which is often ill-defined (see Chapter 1). The development of this behavior has been described postoperatively in patients who binge ate prior to bariatric surgery (Saunders, 2004). This behavior also seems to overlap with "nibbling" or "frequent snacking"—other problems that have been described by various authors (Brolin et al., 1994; Busetto et al., 2002; Saunders, 2004). Saunders (2004) defined *grazing* as a "pattern of repeated episodes of consumption of smaller quantities of food over a longer period of time with accompanying feelings of loss of control" (p. 99). She reported that the majority of patients who engage in such behaviors prior to surgery frequently redevelop such problems after surgery. Bussetto and colleagues (2002) described *nibbling* in 43% of 260 presurgery patients, and Brolin and colleagues suggested that "frequent snacking" preoperatively was associated with attenuated weight loss postoperatively. The lack of valid and reliable instruments to diagnose such problems remains problematic.

At this point there is a lack of agreement as to how to deal with patients who clearly have eating problems that include binge eating, and who may meet criteria for BED, prior to surgery. A recent survey by Devlin and colleagues (2004) speaks to the lack of consensus in this regard. Overall 20% of surgeons indicated that they would proceed with surgery; 27.3% indicated that they would defer surgery; 2.7% indicated that they would not do the surgery, and 50% indicated that they varied the decision based on the individual case.

In the short term there is clear consensus that bariatric surgery can "cure" binge eating, at least for a period of time (Dymek et al., 2001; Kalarchian et al., 1999; Powers et al., 1999). This temporary cure is probably attributable to the fact that following bariatric surgery procedures, most patients are physically unable to consume large amounts of food due to the mechanical limitations on food intake. Given this reality, some researchers have focused on the sense of loss of control rather than objective overeating as the essential diagnostic criteria for problematic binge eating postoperatively. Using this modified definition, there is growing evidence that binge eating may reemerge following surgery, perhaps increasing in prevalence 2 years or more after the operative procedure (Hsu et al., 1996, 1998, 2002; Kalarchian et al., 2002; Lang et al., 2002; Mitchell et al., 2001; Pekkarinen et al., 1994). Work by our group, assessing patients' status 13–15 years postgastric bypass, found that although 49% of patients admitted to binge eating prior to surgery, only 6.4% met criteria for BED at follow-up. However, all those who met criteria for binge eating at follow-up had met criteria for BED prior to surgery, and the recurrence was associated with increased weight regain. In a subsequent cross-sectional study of patients postgastric bypass, 14% patients up to 1 year after surgery, 28% more than 1–

2 years after surgery and 44% more than 2–3 years after surgery reported subjective binge-eating episodes—again suggesting an increased problem with loss of control the more distant the surgery experience (deZwaan et al., 2007).

Overall, there is evidence that binge-eating behavior that is present presurgery is not a strong predictor of attenuated weight loss or weight regain after surgery. However, the reemergence of binge eating or BED, most appropriately defined by a sense of loss of control, is a predictor of less weight loss and/or more weight regain (see Table 5.2).

For example, in our study (Mitchell et al, 2001), patients who developed problems with binge-eating behavior postsurgery experienced substantially more weight regain—a result that was also reported by Kalarchian and colleagues (2002) and Hsu and colleagues (1996). There is

TABLE 5.2. Weight Regain after Surgery and Binge Eating/BED

Authors (year)	Site	Procedure	N	Follow-up (X)	Pre-BE/BED predicts weight loss/regain	Post-BE/BED correlates with weight loss/regain
Rowston et al. (1992)	London	BPD	16	2 yr	—	Yes
Pekkarinen et al. (1994)	Helsinki	VBG	27	5.4 yr	—	Yes
Busetto et al. (1996)	Padova	RYGBP	80	12 mo	No	—
Hsu et al. (1996)	Tufts	VBG	24	3.5 yr	No	Yes
Hsu et al. (1997)	Tufts	RYGBP	27	21 mo	Yes	—
Powers et al. (1999)	University of South Florida	"Gastric restriction"	72	5.5 yr	No	—
Dymek et al. (2001)	University of Chicago	RYGBP	32	6 mo	Yes	—
Mitchell et al. (2001)	Neuropsychiatric Research Institute	RYGBP	78	14 yr	—	Yes
Busetto et al. (2005)	Padova	Lap band	260	3 yr	No	—
Kalarchian et al. (2002)	University of Pittsburgh	RYGBP	99	2–7 yr	—	Yes
Sabbioni et al. (2002)	Bern	VBG	82	2 yr	No	—
Guisado & Vaz (2003)	University of Extramadura (Spain)	VBG	140	18 mo	—	Yes
Boan et al. (2004)	Duke	RYGBP	40	6 mo	No	—
Larsen et al. (2004)	Utrecht	Lap band	160	>2 yr	—	Yes
Malone & Alger-Mayer (2004)	Albany	RYGBP	109	12 mo	No	—
Burgmer et al. (2005)	Essen	Lap band	118	12 mo	No	Yes (sweet eating)
Busetto et al. (2005)	Padova	Lap band	379	5 yr	No	—
Bocchieri-Ricciardi et al. (2006)	University of Chicago	RYGBP	72	m: 18 mo	No	—

Note. BE, binge eating; BED, binge-eating disorder; BPD, biliopancreatic diversion; UBG, vertical-banded gastroplasty; RYGBP, roux-en-Y gastric bypass; lap band, laproscopic banding.

also some evidence that the recurrence of night eating syndrome and other patterns of nocturnal eating may contribute to weight regain (Hsu et al., 1996, 1997; Powers et al., 1999).

Summary

Many patients who are candidates for bariatric surgery have problems with binge eating, and some meet full criteria for BED. There is currently a lack of consensus as to how to deal with these patients. In the short run bariatric surgery procedures seem to eliminate the problem of binge eating. However, over time there is evidence that patients who report subjective overeating and a sense of loss of control—many of whom have had eating problems prior to surgery—will experience less weight loss or more weight regain, and therefore may experience less benefit from bariatric surgery procedures.

This undesirable outcome raises the possibility that some sort of psychosocial intervention could be used to prepare patients who have had problems with binge eating, or BED prior to surgery and are at risk for redeveloping such problems postoperatively. Whether such an intervention should precede or follow surgery, during the period when such problems are most likely to recur—perhaps 18 months to 3 years postsurgery—is unclear. Although some psychological interventions for bariatric surgery patients have been described in the literature (Myers, 2005), including some that address binge eating, there have been no systematic trials of preventive interventions, and no manual-based interventions have been described, although some are now under development. In the next chapter, we review the literature on the psychotherapy of BED, and in Part II we present a detailed CBT treatment manual for BED.

CHAPTER 6

Psychotherapy for Binge-Eating Disorder

Investigators over the past decade have explored a number of distinct psychotherapeutic approaches to the treatment of BED. This chapter reviews the rationale for the various different forms of psychotherapy that have been advanced and summarizes the existing literature regarding their effectiveness. Studies of treatments primarily directed toward weight control that have (in some cases) included comparisons of efficacy in obese binge, versus non-binge, eaters have been discussed elsewhere in this volume (see Chapter 3) and are not reviewed in detail here.

As is illustrated in Figure 6.1, BED is a complex disorder with many contributing factors. The various forms of psychotherapy for BED are based on theories regarding the factors that maintain binge eating. It is worth noting that that the efficacy of a treatment does not necessarily prove the validity of the theory that underlies it. In fact, whereas much research has been conducted regarding treatment response, there have been very few studies of the mechanisms of treatment. Thus, questions regarding *why* treatments work must await the next generation of studies, which will investigate moderators and mediators of response and, perhaps, underlying psychological and physiological mechanisms. The fact that several different approaches to the treatment of binge eating seem to be relatively successful, at least in the short term, raises interesting questions regarding the importance of specific versus nonspecific therapeutic factors.

Figure 6.1 includes obesity in the mix of factors that contribute to the onset and maintenance of BED. Although not all individuals with BED are overweight or obese, most who present for treatment are obese (see Chapter 3), and those of normal weight may nonetheless have significant weight and/or shape concerns. Substituting "subjective obesity"—that is, actual weight higher than one's preferred weight—may render the figure more applicable to those of objectively normal weight. The figure does not include all possible connections between putative binge-promoting factors, but it does suggest the ways in which several factors may interact in mutually reinforcing ways.

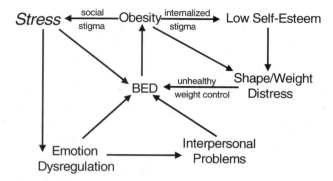

FIGURE 6.1. Psychological and psychosocial factors contributing to the onset and/or maintenance of BED.

Several of the factors in the model have been discussed in greater detail elsewhere in this volume. The association between BED and obesity and the evidence that bears on the possible causal pathways underlying this relationship are summarized in Chapter 3. One of the firmest findings regarding BED is that affected individuals have more Axis I and Axis II psychiatric disorders than weight-matched non–binge eaters (see Chapter 2) and, as such, may have more difficulty regulating their emotions, tolerating distress, and managing their relationships in the stress-filled environment with which most people are, at least intermittently, faced. The Session-by-Session Therapist Guidelines in Part II describe in detail a theoretical model of the psychological factors that lead to and maintain binge eating, including the link between psychological reactivity and binge eating, and the resulting struggle for competence and control.

Psychotherapeutic Approaches to BED

This section briefly describes the various forms of psychotherapy that have been advanced for BED, the principles upon which they are based, and the procedures that are used to address binge eating and related symptoms. Following this, available information concerning the efficacy of each of the treatment approaches is reviewed. As detailed below, different models of psychotherapy for BED focus on different pieces of the BED puzzle.

Cognitive-Behavioral Therapy

The treatment approach that has been best studied to date is CBT. Based on CBT for BN (Fairburn et al., 1993), CBT for BED focuses on the ways in which excessive body shape and weight concern promotes binge eating, and the extreme valuation of shape and weight as a basis for one's self-esteem. Adaptations of CBT for individuals with BED have been outlined in reviews (Devlin, 2001; Marcus, 1997; Pike et al., 2004). In contrast to individuals with BN, those with BED do not typically undereat early in the day and then lose control and binge-eat. But, like those with BN, many individuals with BED do have strict rules about what they are "allowed" to eat. However, they find themselves in violation of these rules much of the time, except when they are in a period of strict dieting and weight loss. It is not surprising that individuals with BED tend to be "yo-yo" dieters, exhibiting frequent weight loss and regain (Spitzer et al., 1992). CBT for BED attempts to help the binge eater normalize her or his eating by adopting a more flexible, healthier eating pattern, loosening the connection between self-esteem and body shape/weight, finding other sources of support for self-esteem, and accepting a larger-than-average body size. As interpreted by most practitioners, this approach does not mean that individuals with BED should avoid weight loss, but rather that this goal should be seen as an outcome of healthy lifestyle changes rather than a prerequisite for self-regard, and perhaps should be deferred until the binge-eating behavior has come under control. The cognitive portion of CBT for BED focuses on increasing consciousness of the links between thoughts, feelings, and behaviors associated with binge eating and acquiring tools to restructure thinking in binge-prone situations.

Because CBT is the most supported psychotherapy for BED, we provide a description of the important components of CBT, whether offered in a group or individual format. A more detailed description of how these components are operationalized in a time-limited treatment program are provided in the treatment program for BED in Part II of this book. The essential elements of CBT for BED follows.

Collaboratively Derived Goals for Change and Self-Acceptance

As discussed in Chapter 3, most individuals who present for treatment of BED manifest somatic (i.e., obesity), behavioral (i.e., binge eating), and psychological (i.e., weight- and shape-related distress, frequent psychiatric comorbidity) symptoms. It is crucial for therapist and patient to discuss these features of the disorder, agree on treatment priorities, and, if there is more than one goal, the order in which the goals will be pursued. In particular, CBT, as it is usually practiced, does not initially emphasize weight loss but rather is focused on reducing and eliminating binge eating and promoting a balance of healthy change and self-acceptance. In light of the prominent stigmatization of obesity in our culture, combined with patients' prior experience with weight loss programs, it can be difficult for patients and their families to grasp these priorities. Although patients generally do not wish to give up the goal of weight loss (nor should they, from a heath-promotion point of view), they are often amenable to deferring weight loss goals until their eating is better controlled, and to focusing on long-term weight management rather than short-term weight loss. For patients whose primary desire is to lose weight as rapidly as possible, CBT is probably not an ideal treatment choice.

Coherent Client-Specific Model for the Maintenance of BED

As is the case when beginning CBT for any disorder, it is useful for therapist and patient to jointly develop an explicit model of the factors responsible for the maintenance of the disorder and how they interact. Figure 6.1 illustrates one such model. This type of diagram is useful not only because it aids our understanding of how the disorder is maintained, but also because it provides a "road map" for treatment, suggesting the various dimensions of the disorder that must be addressed in order to begin to undermine the system that maintains binge eating and ensure the maintenance of this change. It is important that this model is tailored to the particular patient and that it is seen as a "work in progress" that can be amended and expanded over the course of treatment. This issue is addressed in more detail in Part II, which emphasizes the need to obtain a great deal of self-report data from each patient, to help the therapist understand any given individual's problems.

Education and Healthy Lifestyle Counseling

Education, either via oral explanation or the provision of written materials, is a crucial component of treatment. Early in treatment, it is particularly useful for the patient to begin to understand the multiple causes of obesity, including genetic, biological, and environmental causes. Patients entering treatment often subscribe to the "willpower" theory of obesity—that is, that they are to blame for their obesity because they lack the will or strength to change. It can be tremendously relieving for patients to realize that, in fact, the task of losing weight and maintaining weight loss for someone who is predisposed to obesity is extremely difficult, particularly in an obesity-promoting environment. At the same time, it is important for the therapist *not* to convey that change is impossible, but rather that the patient deserves credit for any amount of change she or he is able to achieve and maintain. Many of the readings and forms that patients are asked to complete in Part II can be seen as psychoeducational. CBT frequently involves a heavy reliance on homework readings and assignment, in some ways reminiscent of classwork rather than traditional psychodynamic psychotherapy. This strategy allows the therapist to expand the therapy into the patient's daily life, and it also allows for far more material to be covered than would otherwise be possible. When used correctly, these forms prompt patients to reflect on their own situation—a particularly important component in group therapy, wherein individual attention from the therapist is more limited.

Patients also benefit from basic nutritional education, including the relative health-promoting effects of various food choices, not limited simply to caloric values, and principles of healthier eating (e.g., checking food labels; consuming adequate amounts of vegetables, fruits, and fiber; minimizing consumption of saturated fats and trans fatty acids). In addition, exercise counseling that is geared to what is realistic for the patient and includes lifestyle exercise (i.e., exercise as part of one's daily routine, like using the stairs instead of the elevator or walking rather than driving to work) as well as programmed exercise is key.

Self-Monitoring

Self-monitoring is a core component of CBT for most disorders. In the case of BED, it generally takes the form of keeping food diaries and recording binge-eating episodes, including associated circumstances, feelings, and thoughts. Generally these records do not entail counting calories, at least at the outset of treatment. For many patients, the calorie-counting pattern tends to promote the overly restrictive "dietetic" eating behaviors that they have undertaken in the past, usually then lapsing into a period of insufficient dietary restraint and binge eating. The goal is for patients to develop a flexible but consistent pattern of eating that is realistic for long-term maintenance, and, of course, to eliminate binge eating and other unhealthy eating patterns. Self-monitoring forms are included in Part II; their use should be heavily emphasized early in treatment, when adherence to such tasks may be limited.

Behavioral Tools

Behavioral tools are based on well-established behavioral principles—that is, on the identification of links between conditioned stimuli and unwanted responses, and the reinforcement of desired responses. For example, stimulus control techniques include limiting one's exposure to binge-prone environments—for example, avoiding all-you-can-eat buffets, asking the waiter to remove the bread basket, or keeping food-filled serving dishes off the table. Healthy eating and activity patterns can be reinforced with planned rewards (e.g., pleasant relaxation with a friend after biking or jogging together). In particular, binge-eating episodes are analyzed to determine the chain of events ("behavior chain") that led to the eating binge, and various "link-breaking" techniques are explored that might limit exposure to the relevant cues or reinforce healthier behaviors in similar situations. Readings and forms to educate patients about these issues and record data regarding their own eating behaviors are included in Part II.

Cognitive Tools

Cognitive tools include both motivational techniques, such as decision analysis, and change-focused techniques, such as cognitive restructuring. *Decision analysis* refers to the identification of two mutually exclusive choices—for example, "I will work on breaking out of the cycle of dieting and binge eating" versus "I will continue to undertake new diets that might help me rapidly lose the weight I want to lose"—and the systematic exploration of the pros and cons, both in the short and long term, of these two options. This technique can be extremely helpful in revealing the barriers to change, including the assumptions and possible misconceptions that may be influencing the patient's choice, and in focusing the patient and therapist on the work needed to overcome these obstacles. At the same time, decision analysis can be useful in consolidating the motivation for change by providing a comprehensive list of the potential advantages of change, to which the patient can refer whenever motivation begins to flag.

Cognitive restructuring is at the core of CBT for BED. This technique involves mapping the circumstances, automatic thoughts, and feelings that lead to binge eating, and systematically attempting to recognize and reconsider those automatic thoughts in ways that alter feelings and behavior (binge eating). Cognitive restructuring often leads to the identification of deeply held beliefs about oneself or one's interaction with the world, associated with feelings, memories, and somatic sensations that may be activated in various situations. The identification of such core beliefs, or schemas, and recognition of how they influence one's interpretation of various situations or circumstances can be extremely useful—despite the fact that schemas are often quite resistant to change. Again, cognitive restructuring is an important element in the Part II program. This technique is a difficult challenge for some patients, and patients who are particularly concrete in their thinking may only master it superficially at best. In such cases other strategies should be emphasized.

An important point regarding cognitive restructuring with individuals who are overweight or obese is that the realities of living in a fat-phobic society must be recognized and addressed. Nonetheless, patients may have skewed interpretations of the relationship between cultural values and individual experience. For example, the fact that society, as a whole, prefers thinner body types does not imply that no one will be attracted to someone who does not fit the cultural ideal. For some patients, the commitment to health and acceptance at any size and the idea of working for change not just on an individual but also on a societal level can energize treatment and strengthen motivation.

Experiential Learning/Behavioral Experiments

Although cognitive tools can be quite useful in beginning to undermine the assumptions and maladaptive patterns in which the patient is mired, experiential learning—that is, the disconfirmation of previously held predictions—is probably the most powerful teacher. For example, a patient who avoids taking a dance class because she is convinced that she will be entirely inept and that her body will be ridiculed by others may undertake the experiment of signing up for such a class, thereby creating the possibility that her prediction can be disconfirmed. A patient who is convinced that she can no longer ride a bicycle may find that, with practice, she is able not only to ride as she once did, but actually enjoys doing so. A patient who believes that he will not be able to relax and unwind unless he eats a pint of ice cream while watching the news may find that a bowl of fruit, eaten mindfully before or following the news, works just as well.

Relapse Prevention

Because binge eating tends to be a recurring problem, it is important that patients leave treatment with the necessary tools to manage their vulnerability to binge eating and to respond rapidly and effectively to lapses. A comprehensive relapse prevention plan includes both a set of daily practices to maintain health and a detailed plan for dealing with the slips that inevitably occur. An additional element of relapse prevention is the anticipation of possible binge-promoting situations (e.g., going on a cruise) and the construction, in advance, of a plan to minimize risk. Isolation is often an important element of the road to relapse; group support, therefore, can exert a powerful protective influence. Further details on these and other elements of CBT for BED can be found in Part II of this book.

Interpersonal Therapy

An interesting alternative approach to the treatment of BED is IPT, originally developed as a treatment for depression and later adapted by Fairburn and colleagues for eating disorders (as noted in Weissman et al., 2000). Although IPT was originally developed as an individual psychotherapy, the form of IPT that has been most studied for patients with BED is an IPT adapted for a group context. A comprehensive description of IPT tailored for a group setting can be found in Wilfley and colleagues (2000b).

As adapted for BED, IPT works with individuals to identify interpersonal problem areas that seem to be most closely linked to the maintenance of binge eating. Interpersonal history and context of binge-eating episodes are analyzed for evidence of problems in one or more of four areas of interpersonal functioning: (1) unresolved grief, (2) role transition (e.g., moving into or out of a marriage), (3) role dispute (e.g., a breakdown in communication with a significant other), and (4) interpersonal deficit (i.e., a pervasive and long-standing difficulty initiating or maintaining relationships). The focus in IPT is to begin to make progress in the interpersonal problem area and find new ways of improving the situation and/or moving on, thereby undermining the system that maintained binge eating and paving the way for change.

Dialectical Behavior Therapy

Dialectical behavior therapy (DBT) was originally developed for individuals with borderline personality disorder as a means of managing unbearable emotional states that lead to self-destructive behavior (Linehan, 1993a, 1993b). DBT training typically involves four modules: mindfulness skills, distress tolerance, emotion regulation, and interpersonal management strategies. DBT is often administered in a group setting, and as it is adapted for BED (Wiser & Telch, 1999), it is a pragmatic, skills-oriented treatment that provides the participant with concrete skills that can be used in distressing, binge-prone situations.

A related form of treatment for BED is mindfulness meditation, which is designed to help individuals cope with various forms of stress and psychological or physical pain that, if unchecked, may lead to binge eating. Mindfulness, as conceptualized by practitioners such as Kabat-Zinn (1990), refers to the attempt to direct one's attention to the present moment and to maintain a focused, detached, and nonjudgmental awareness and acceptance of both one's internal states and one's environment, rather than attempting to fight off, or becoming overwhelmed by, these conditions. Mindfulness is a practice that can be learned and cultivated; it has been found to be useful in managing stress in a variety of contexts, including medical and psychiatric illness.

Behavioral Weight Control Treatment

Treatment approaches that emphasize healthy lifestyle change, along with low-calorie diet (LCD) or VLCD, with the primary goal of weight loss, without particular attention to binge eating, have also been used with obese binge eaters who meet BED criteria. Behavioral weight control approaches, as outlined in the LEARN manual (Brownell, 2007), for example, take a psychoeducational approach to topics of lifestyle, exercise, attitudes, relationships, and nutrition, with the goal of helping patients develop and maintain healthier patterns. As summarized in Chapter 3, there is some evidence that, at least for subjects who present to weight control programs, such approaches can be equally helpful for binge and non–binge eaters. Fewer studies have examined behavioral weight control approaches specifically for patients with BED, with the primary goal of cessation of binge eating but with weight loss as an important additional goal. The goals of such treatment are to optimize weight loss and maintenance of lower weight while, at the same time, helping patients maintain long-term remission of binge eating.

Summary of Treatment Approaches

The interesting conclusion that can be drawn from the various psychotherapeutic approaches that have been developed for BED is that the complex configuration of interlocking factors that maintains BED can be disrupted at several different points. Clinicians often note that individuals who begin to improve in one area that has been particularly targeted in their treatment (e.g., interpersonal relationships) may spontaneously make improvements in other areas of functioning (e.g., self-acceptance, healthy lifestyle, stress management). However, this does not suggest that treatments are interchangeable; further research may provide a rational basis for matching particular treatments to particular individuals, depending on their specific goals and clinical features.

Studies of Psychotherapy for BED

The following section selectively reviews the controlled studies of psychotherapy for BED that have been conducted to date, particularly including moderate-to-large-scale studies using DSM-IV-TR Appendix B criteria for BED (American Psychiatric Association, 2000). Table 6.1 summarizes outcomes in the major studies using psychotherapy for patients with BED, with binge abstinence as the primary goal of treatment.

As can be seen from Table 6.1, a variety of psychotherapeutic approaches, including CBT, IPT, psychodynamic interpersonal therapy (PIP), DBT, and BWL are effective in bringing about short-term remission of binge eating in a substantial proportion of individuals with BED. Follow-up data over periods up to 12 months suggest variable maintenance of improvement, with most studies reporting continued improvement from baseline, but several studies showing significant deterioration from the posttreatment assessment.

No treatments other than BWL have yet been found to bring about significant weight reduction, and the results from studies of BWL in this group (i.e., patients presenting primarily for treatment of binge eating as opposed to weight loss) are variable. The study of Nauta and colleagues (2000) reported a statistically and clinically significant weight loss in patients receiving BWL at posttreatment, but weight was regained at 6-month follow-up. In the study of Agras and colleagues (1994), subjects receiving BWL—particularly those who also received desipramine, showed some weight loss at 3-month follow-up. An additional study (Reeves et al., 2001) using BWL found significant reduction in binge eating but no weight loss in subjects receiving BWL, and the same group, in a separate study, reported that neither dieting nor nondieting treatment yielded significant weight loss in overweight women with binge eating (Goodrick et al., 1998). In a recent study, a self-help version of BWL did not yield significant weight reduction in individuals with BED (Grilo & Masheb, 2005). A preliminary report from this same group suggested that neither group BWL nor group CBT yielded clinically significant weight loss in obese patients with BED, and CBT was superior to BWL in reducing binge eating (Grilo et al., 2006). In a 1-year follow-up study of patients with BED who had received CBT followed by BWL (Agras et al., 1997), participants were found to maintain reductions in binge eating reasonably well, but changes in weight were neither significant nor sustained. However, the subgroup of patients who achieved binge abstinence did show significant sustained weight loss, suggesting that binge cessation may lead to a more favorable weight course in these patients. Further evidence that binge abstinence may lead to weight stabilization, as opposed to ongoing weight gain in those who continue to binge eat, is summarized in Chapter 3. Consistent with this finding, an early study suggested that, in order to optimize weight loss, the severity of binge eating must be taken into account, as women with more severe binge eating lost more weight in a treatment tailored to binge eating, whereas women with only moderate binge eating did better using a standard BWL approach (Porzelius et al., 1995). This finding suggests that severity rather than simply the presence or absence of binge eating may importantly influence treatment outcome and differential response to treatment approaches.

In light of the fact that an initial course of psychotherapy does not lead to binge abstinence in all individuals with BED, some investigators have examined possible next steps in treatment

TABLE 6.1. Selected Controlled Studies of Psychotherapy for BED

Authors (year)	N randomized (completed)	Treatments	Format	Percent binge abstinent[a]	Comments
Telch et al. (1990)	23 (17) 21 (15)	CBT WLC	Group	79% 0%	Nonpurging BN. 1-week abstinence. Completers. 36% CBT abstinent at 10-week F/U.
Agras et al. (1994)	36 (30) 37 (27)	CBT/BWL BWL	Group	37% 19%	1-week abstinence. Completers. 28% CBT/BWL and 14% BWL abstinent at 3-month F/U.
Nauta et al. (2000)	21 (18) 16 (13)	CBT BWL	Group	67% 44%	86% CBT and 44% BWL abstinent at 6-month F/U.
Peterson et al. (1998)	16 (14) 19 (17) 15 (11) 11 (9)	CBT CBT/GSH CBT/PSH WLC	Group	68.8% 68.4% 86.7% 12.5%	1-week abstinence.
Carter & Fairburn (1998)	34 (26) 35 (34) 24 (23)	CBT/GSH CBT/PSH WLC	Individual	50% 43% 8%	50% CBT/GSH and 40% CBT/PSH abstinent at 6-month F/U.
Grilo & Masheb (2005)	37 (32) 38 (25) 15 (13)	CBT/GSH BWL/GSH ATC	Individual	59.5% 23.7% 26.7%	
Wilfley et al. (1993)	18 (12) 18 (16) 20 (19)	CBT IPT WLC	Group	28% 44% 0%	Nonpurging BN. 1-week abstinence.
Wilfley et al. (2002)	81 (78) 81 (80)	CBT IPT	Group	82% 74%	Completers. 72% CBT and 70% IPT abstinent at 12-month F/U.
Telch et al. (2001)	22 (18) 22 (16)	DBT WLC	Group	89% 12.5%	Completers. DBT: 56% abstinent at 6-month F/U.
Tasca et al. (2006)	47 (37) 48 (37) 40 (33)	CBT PIP WLC	Group	62.2% 59.5% 12.1%	1-week abstinence. Completers. 67.7% CBT and 56.8% PIP abstinent at 12-month F/U.

Note. CBT, cognitive-behavioral therapy; WLC, wait-list control; BWL, behavioral weight loss; GSH, guided self-help; PSH, pure self-help; ATC, attentional control; IPT, interpersonal therapy; DBT, dialectical behavior therapy; PIP, psychodynamic interpersonal therapy; BN, bulimia nervosa; F/U, follow-up.

[a]Abstinence rates in randomized sample, except as noted in Comments (completers). Abstinence rates pertain to 28-day recall, except as noted in Comments (1-week abstinence).

and their efficacy for those who did not respond to the initial treatment. Agras and colleagues (1995) found that a course of group IPT did not lead to further improvement in individuals who failed to improve with an initial course of group CBT. A subsequent study from the same group (Eldredge et al., 1997) found that extending a 12-week course of group CBT for BED by adding an additional 12 sessions appeared to be helpful for individuals who initially did not respond to treatment. Pendleton and colleagues (2002) similarly found that extending group CBT for BED by adding a 6-month maintenance phase yielded additional clinical benefit. Further study of secondary interventions for nonresponders is clearly needed. However, a preliminary conclusion that can be drawn from these initial studies is that the duration of treatment may importantly influence the proportion of individuals who will ultimately respond to treatment. Thus, in comparing treatment response across studies, it is important to consider the possible effect of length of treatment as one of several factors that may account for observed differences.

Another group of studies has taken a different approach to the problem of incomplete response to treatment by examining the utility of various treatment augmentation strategies. The provision of structured exercise in the form of fitness instruction and gym membership has been found to significantly augment the clinical benefits of group CBT for BED (Pendleton et al., 2002). In contrast, involving spouses in group CBT by having them attend group meetings and encouraging them to actively partner with patients in further healthy lifestyle changes did not yield additional benefit (Gorin et al., 2003). Similarly, the use of an ecological momentary assessment system for self-monitoring, in which patients complete pocket diaries, noting circumstances, mood, and other experiences both at mealtimes and when signaled by a programmable wristwatch, did not appear to effectively add to the benefit of CBT for BED (le Grange et al., 2002). Devlin and colleagues (2005) recently reported that adding individual CBT to group BWL for obese individuals with BED significantly augmented binge reduction. Further studies of such combined interventions, including their cost effectiveness, are warranted.

An additional strategy for enhancing psychotherapy for BED is to attempt to change attitudes toward body image using exposure-based techniques. Hilbert and colleagues (2002) have reported preliminary findings suggesting that body image exposure using mirror confrontation may, in the short term, led to a reduction in negative cognitions and improvement in appearance self-esteem. A virtual-reality-based treatment using a computer-based immersive virtual reality system to address eating control, body image, and managing a variety of social environments has been found to be a promising method of operationalizing CBT for BED in women participating in a residential weight control program (Riva et al., 2002, 2003). This innovative approach to treating BED is one that merits further study.

Additional studies that fall under the rubric of augmentation treatments have addressed the temporal continuum of treatment and the different stages at which interventions may be helpful. Dunn and colleagues (2006) studied the possible utility of a single session of motivational enhancement therapy (MET) as a lead-in to self-help CBT treatment for binge eating (full threshold or subthreshold BN or BED). Although they found that the MET session yielded increased readiness for change, they were unable to detect effects on target symptoms following self-help treatment. Further investigation of MET will be needed to fully understand its possible utility in the treatment of BED and related conditions. Another possible role for CBT would be to minimize relapse, particularly breakthrough binge eating, following a weight loss intervention in patients with BED. A study conducted by de Zwaan and colleagues (2005a) reported that, whereas the overall effectiveness of a VLCD program for obese women with BED was comparable to that of other treatments for BED and additionally yielded significant weight loss that was partially maintained at 1-year follow-up, the addition of a CBT component during the last 12 weeks of the program did not improve results. These studies underscore the importance of considering the various time points in treatment at which additional interventions may confer additional clinical benefit.

Studies of Psychotherapy and Medication for BED

A final set of studies has employed combinations of medication and psychotherapy in the treatment of obese individuals with BED. Four studies (Devlin et al., 2005; Grilo et al., 2005b; Molinari et al., 2005; Ricca et al., 2001) examined the utility of fluoxetine, CBT, and the combination of the two. The studies differed somewhat in design, with one study (Devlin et al., 2005) examining individual CBT and fluoxetine treatments as add-ons to group BWL, and one study (Molinari et al., 2005) implementing treatment initially in an inpatient setting. Despite these differences in design, the studies are impressively consistent in suggesting that CBT is more effective than fluoxetine in the treatment of BED, and that fluoxetine treatment adds little or no additional benefit. One study (Devlin et al., 2005) found that fluoxetine treatment was associated with greater reduction in depressive symptoms but not with reduction in binge eating. The study of Ricca and colleagues (2001) suggested that fluvoxamine, but not fluoxetine, might enhance the effect of CBT on binge eating.

In contrast to the apparently limited utility of adding fluoxetine to psychotherapy for BED, two studies (Agras et al., 1994; Laederach-Hofmann et al., 1999) suggest that adding tricyclic antidepressant treatment to a course of BWL and/or CBT/BWL, or diet counseling may confer additional clinical benefit. The study of Agras and colleagues (1994) found that desipramine did not add to the initial effectiveness of BWL or CBT/BWL, either in terms of binge reduction or weight loss, but that medication seemed to be associated with additional weight loss at 3-month posttreatment follow-up. Laederach-Hofmann and colleagues (1999) reported that patients receiving an initial 8-week treatment with imipramine combined with diet counseling and psychological support, followed by 6 months of continued counseling without medication, showed greater weight loss and greater improvement in depressive symptoms at the end of the 6-month maintenance period than patients who received the identical treatment but without medication during the initial 8 weeks. Most recently, Grilo and colleagues (2005a) have reported that orlistat, a lipase inhibitor that blocks the absorption of dietary fat, added to CBT guided self-help, significantly augmented weight loss in obese binge eaters.

Summary

Although many different approaches to psychotherapy for BED have been pioneered over the last two decades and several systematic studies have been conducted, a great deal is still unknown. At this point, we can conclude that several different psychotherapeutic approaches are effective in reducing or eliminating binge eating in some, but not all, individuals with BED, at least in the short term, with variable response during the year following treatment.

Factors such as the level of binge eating of participants, the treatment setting, and the duration of treatment are important in interpreting the results of psychotherapy studies. Further studies of treatment combinations, novel approaches to treatment or to augmenting standard treatments, and psychotherapeutic interventions at different stages of treatment are all greatly needed. In addition, although initial studies of adding fluoxetine to CBT for BED have not supported its routine use in this setting, the available studies of combined medication and psychotherapy for BED are still very limited, and it is too early to draw any overall conclusion with confidence regarding the utility of combined treatment for BED.

CHAPTER 7

Binge-Eating Disorder and the Future

As this text is being finalized, plans are underway for the development of the Eating Disorders Task Force for DSM-V, which is now targeted for publication in 2011. There are obviously a number of issues that will face this task force, but one of the most prominent will be the status of BED in the next revision of the nomenclature. Despite the fact that BED was not given full status in DSM-IV, a large research literature has accumulated on this condition, suggesting that it is a clinically meaningful form of psychopathology that is accompanied by impairment and decreased quality of life, and clearly is worthy of serious consideration for full status.

BED must be regarded in the context of other issues regarding EDNOS. Exactly what is the relationship between BED and obesity? This question is addressed in detail in the text, but a number of other questions have been raised that need to be addressed in subsequent studies. Although BED is associated with distress and impairment in its own right, to the degree to which it contributes to the onset, persistence, progression, or impact of obesity, it takes on an even greater public health significance. Also, it isn't clear how other possible pieces of EDNOS, such as the night eating syndrome and the proposed purging disorder, will be addressed as well.

As mentioned in the text, loss of control around eating and binge-eating episodes are clearly seen in childhood and adolescence and appear to be a risk factor for the development of obesity. Very little research has been done in this area, but existing findings suggest that this area is of great public health importance, and additional resources need to be directed to examining binge eating in childhood and adolescence. The available literature also suggests that there may be different routes to the development of BED, ranging from uncontrolled eating prior to the onset of obesity to dietary restriction in the context of obesity. This area also needs to be examined in larger samples, particularly in terms of prediction of treatment response.

What we know about binge eating in the context of BED suggests that there are significant similarities but also important differences in eating behavior between BED and BN. In particular, the eating binges in BED tend to last longer and to be smaller relative to kilocalories consumed. However, many questions remain regarding the microstructure of binge eating, precipitants and sequelae of binge eating in BED, and further work in this area is needed. In addition, differences in binge eating at a phenomenological level may be indicative of differences in underlying pathophysiological mechanisms and may spur further investigation of these differences.

The issues of comorbidity, which are also outlined in the text, raise intriguing questions regarding the relationship of BED to other forms of psychopathology. In particular, the relationships between BED and mood disorders, anxiety disorders, alcohol/substance use/abuse disorders need further examination. A better understanding of this comorbidity may have important implications both for clinical care and for our understanding of the etiology and psychobiology of BED.

The psychobiology of BED is just now beginning to be addressed. We know that binge eating is a highly heritable behavior, and the available studies suggest that BED does cluster in families. Therefore, because there is a strong possibility that genetic factors are involved in the development of BED, this area clearly needs to be examined further in the years ahead. Furthermore, changes in the gastric functioning of patients with BED suggest the possibility that other systems involved in the control of appetite and satiety may also be abnormal. This area also needs to be explored further. As the number of biological factors that are implicated in the control of appetite and satiety grows, they will need to be examined in patients with BED.

What little is available relative to cultural factors suggests that there are large differences between different groups, and although the epidemiological studies on cultural differences have been small in number to date, this clearly is an area where expanded research is necessary. To a large extent, eating behavior is culturally determined, and it must be assumed that such would be true about the phenomenon of binge eating in patients with BED.

Another issue concerns physician education. Obesity has moved into the forefront of concern for many primary care providers, but the role of BED specifically and binge eating more broadly also needs to be at the forefront of the consciousness of physicians who work with obese patients, because BED may be a treatable phenomenon that may impact the course of obesity.

The treatment literature continues to evolve. Our psychotherapy approaches, including CBT, appear to be quite effective in eliminating or suppressing binge eating but usually do not result in substantial weight loss. The pharmacotherapy approaches also appear promising, and some of these have been associated with more substantial weight loss—but exactly how to package interventions for both weight loss and binge-eating cessation has not yet been adequately addressed. In addition, very few studies have examined the long-term effects of treatment interventions on the course of BED and obesity. Further combination treatment studies and longer-term studies are clearly indicated for individuals with BED. Identifying individuals at high risk for the development of obesity because of binge-eating behavior in childhood and adolescence and developing structured interventions to address this behavior may offer a very important route toward a means of preventing a subgroup of obesity.

The delineation of BED also has had an interesting effect on the field of eating disorders and the field of obesity. Eating disorder scholars have become more interested in obesity, in general, and obesity researchers have developed a renewed interest in behavior as a risk factor for obesity. This continuing dialogue will strengthen both fields in the years ahead.

PART II

A Cognitive-Behavioral Treatment
Program for Binge-Eating Disorder

Introduction to This Treatment Program

In this second part of the book, we provide a cognitive-behavioral treatment manual for BED. The manual's purpose is to provide guidance to therapists in helping patients overcome problems with BED.

The model used in this approach is a form of CBT that has now been used in two randomized trials, one conducted at the University of Minnesota (Peterson et al., 1998, 2001) and the second conducted at the University of Minnesota and at the Neuropsychiatric Research Institute in Fargo, North Dakota (Peterson et al., 2006). In these trials, the full CBT program was compared to (1) a treatment condition wherein the psychoeducation parts of the sessions were delivered via videotape, with the therapist present during the second half of the session; (2) a treatment condition wherein patients viewed the videotapes, then did self-help using written instructions, and did not see a therapist; and (3) a waiting-list control. At end of treatment, 78.6% of those in the therapist-led condition, 75% in the therapist-assisted condition, and 90% in the self-help condition were no longer binge-eating, compared to 12.5% in the waiting-list group. (There were no statistically significant differences among the treatment groups and all treatments were superior to the waiting-list control condition.) The sample size was modest, with 61 participants. The same four treatments were then used in the second study, which enrolled 259 subjects and utilized more rigorous assessment measures. In this replication study, the rates of abstinence were lower (50% therapist led, 33.3% therapist assisted, 17.9% self-help, 10.1% waiting-list control), with the best results obtained in the therapist-led cell on most variables.

Treatment Goals

The focus of the program is on behavioral change rather than understanding any specific precursor of the illness or any dynamic antecedents. The overall goals include the following:

1. To interrupt binge-eating behavior.
2. To reinstitute more normal eating habits.
3. Whenever possible, to change erroneous beliefs about weight and shape and develop healthier attitudes towards one's body.

Therapist Qualifications

The manual presumes familiarity with CBT techniques as well as some working knowledge of nutrition. The role of the therapist is to actively provide encouragement, support, and information, but the responsibility for change rests firmly with the patient.

Patients Appropriate for This Treatment

This treatment is designed for adults with BED who do not have another type of severe psychopathology that would require additional intervention (e.g., suicidal ideation, psychosis).

Program and Session Structure

The therapy can be conducted in either an individual or group format. The basic structure of the therapy consists of 15 sessions over 20 weeks—10 weeks of weekly sessions, 10 weeks of biweekly sessions. Session length is 45 minutes to an hour in individual therapy and 80–90 minutes in group session. Groups should be closed, with all patients participating in the group from the beginning and no new members admitted along the way. In addition, groups should contain anywhere from 4 to 10 patients, of only one gender, if possible.

There are three phases in the treatment. Phase I (sessions 1–6) teaches behavioral and cognitive strategies that target binge eating. Phase II (sessions 7–13) addresses associated problems that often accompany binge-eating behaviors. Phase III (sessions 14 and 15) focuses on maintaining improvement and preventing relapse. The material covered in Phase I begins with basic information about BED, followed by a delineation of cues and consequences and a careful assessment of the relationships of thoughts, feelings, and behaviors. The sessions then focus on restructuring thoughts and developing strategies for interrupting cues and chains of behavior. In Phase II the therapy shifts to specific areas, including an examination of body image, self-esteem, stress management, problem solving, and assertiveness, as well as weight management. The last two sessions, Phase III, are devoted to relapse prevention.

This CBT approach is highly structured and relies heavily on reading and homework assignments. Subjects are instructed to read materials prior to attending the next session and then are given additional homework assignments to complete before the next session. In general, each session follows a pattern that includes the following elements:

1. Review of the homework from the previous session, including the forms that have been completed.
2. Agenda setting for the current session.

3. Discussion of the new materials; the therapist covers the material and uses information the patient has provided previously or during the session to illustrate the material.
4. Assignment of homework for the next session, including a review of which forms need to be completed and, when indicated, directions as to how to fill out the forms.

In this program, a great deal of material needs to be covered in a relatively short period of time. The therapist should be comfortable lecturing, being directive at times, and keeping the therapy "on track." When patients digress and introduce problems that are not the focus of therapy, whether in an individual therapy or group setting, they may need to be reminded that other problems may require other therapy, perhaps following the current treatment. Not uncommonly, the therapist will need to refocus patients.

Patients should be encouraged to read the materials in the manual several times. They should be instructed to set aside 30–60 minutes each evening to reread previous sessions, focus on those that have been particularly helpful, and read ahead in the manual to cover the material not yet reviewed.

In a therapy approach such as this one, patients initially may resist doing the reading and homework assignments. This resistance should be addressed firmly but nonjudgmentally. Patients need to complete the homework for the therapy to be successful. When at all possible, reward patients verbally for things they have completed. If necessary, allow patients time in the session to complete the needed forms, while mentioning that time devoted to form completion hinders the thrust of therapy and leaves less time for actual discussion.

As is the case with most therapies, patients vary in the degree to which they understand and utilize specific techniques. This variability is perhaps most observable when teaching how to restructure thoughts. Some patients take to this technique readily, finding it very helpful. Others find it particularly challenging and do not really progress far beyond the use of basic behavioral technique because the cognitive issues are too demanding or too confusing. The guiding principle here is to ascertain how much the patient understands and, in particular, what seems to work well for her or him and then to emphasize those techniques. No patient will profit equally from all the skills, and enough are provided that most patients will be able to find several that are useful for them in dealing with their eating disorder on a day-to-day basis.

Conceptual Framework for This Treatment

Patients, like all of us, think about their appearance, health, relationships, interests, abilities, and futures. Their thinking, like everyone's, is prone to error.

The underlying thesis of this treatment program is that misconceptions about food, eating, body weight, and body shape interfere with the patient's efforts to adapt and live securely in the environment. Treatment should provide a clear and relatively consistent framework for helping patients identify, evaluate, and change their inaccurate thoughts and feelings about food and eating, and to learn more adaptive eating behaviors.

For our purposes here, *behavior* can be viewed as consisting of three basic components: a cue, a network of responses, and a consequence. The response network is a complex structure that consists of interacting thoughts, feelings, and behaviors. The cue triggers the response network; consequences follow. In many cases, a consequence can itself become a cue for subse-

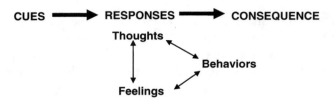

FIGURE II.1. The three basic components of behavior: a triggering cue, a network of responses (interacting thoughts, feelings, and behaviors), and the consequence.

quent responses. Figure II.1 depicts this basic understanding of behavioral components. The following material discusses each component in more detail.

Cues

Cues (also known as antecedents and triggers) are *situations that trigger* the problematic thoughts, feelings, and behaviors—that is, the response network. Examples of cues that often trigger unhealthy eating habits are listed below. Note that cues come from either *internal* or *external* sources.

Internal cues
Cognitive: a memory, a mental picture or image, a wish

Affective: an underlying mood state (e.g., depression, anxiety)

Physiological: physical discomfort; hunger and satiety; activity level (physical exhaustion or inactivity); proprioceptive changes (e.g., feeling too full); metabolic or hormonal changes (e.g., premenstrual bloating, fluid and electrolyte disturbances)

External cues
Social or interpersonal: being with a person who engages in a problem behavior; stimulus from the mass media; extreme sensory stimulation (crowds or isolation)

Environmental: weather (e.g., humidity, temperature); location (at home, work, school; at the ocean, in the mountains; in the city, country; on a plane, boat, in a car; in the living room); extreme sensory stimulation (disorganization or disorder vs. extreme order or monotony)

Specific object: hearing, seeing, smelling, touching, or tasting an object or thing (e.g., seeing an advertisement, smelling a pie, touching money)

The Response Network

Thoughts include ideas, notions, self-statements, expectations, beliefs, and assumptions. Beliefs and assumptions are ideas that are taken for granted and are not questioned. Thoughts operate on two information-processing modes: *automatic* (spontaneous) and *deliberate* (reasoned through).

Feelings encompass both emotional and physiological responses and include hunger pangs and tension; vigor and fatigue; fluctuations in emotions from elation to demoralization and depression, as well as feelings of guilt, shame, apprehension, or joy.

Behaviors refer to the actions the person performs and the words the person says aloud. Facial expressions and other nonverbal behaviors (e.g., agitation, impatience, withdrawal, secrecy) are indications of the response network.

Note in Figure II.1 that thoughts and feelings are aligned vertically. These are the *internal responses* that are often difficult for observers—as well as patients—to infer. One task of the therapeutic process is to help the patient become aware of and identify her or his internal responses to cues. Note also that although behaviors stand to the right of thoughts and feelings in the figure, they could have been placed just as easily to their left. Behaviors are the overt *external responses* that can be identified by observers as well as by patients. Behaviors *interact* with thoughts and feelings. A person's thoughts and feelings affect her or his actions, just as the person's actions affect her or his thoughts and feelings.

Consequences

Consequences are the *conditions that follow* a network of thoughts, feelings, and behaviors. Consequences are basically *positive or negative, immediate and/or delayed*, and *vary in strength*.

Consequences often perceived as positive
Tend to be immediate: feeling satisfied, not hungry; emotional relief; release of physical tension; avoiding difficult or unpleasant situations; not feeling deprived

Tend to be delayed: weight gain, self-reward (purchases); sense of belonging (e.g., related to social eating)

Consequences often perceived as negative
Tend to be immediate: feeling out of control; feeling fat, bloated

Tend to be delayed: depression; weight gain; constipation, bloatedness; jeopardized social relationships and academic/work standing; financial problems; medical problems

Consequences are classified along three dimensions: value, power (salience), and time.

Value: Positive versus Negative

The value dimension refers to how the person perceives a particular consequence and the meaning the person assigns to it. Consequences are generally perceived as basically positive or basically negative. *Positive* consequences are rewarding; they encourage responses to be repeated. *Negative* consequences—*when they are in the person's awareness*—are inhibiting; they encourage a change in responses. Hence, positive consequences maintain behavior, whereas negative consequences alter behavior.

Complexity is introduced into this simple behavioral formula when individual differences are taken into account. One person may perceive a consequence as positive, whereas another may perceive the same consequence as negative. For example:

— Helen may perceive the perspiration from rope jumping as a positive consequence, but Heidi may perceive it as a negative consequence.
— Harold may perceive the tension release from binge eating as positive, but Hank may perceive it as negative.

Patients first need to *become aware* of the consequences of their behavior and then to label each consequence as either positive or negative.

Power: More versus Less

Even when a person is aware of a negative consequence, that consequence may not have sufficient power to overcome a competing, positive consequence and to influence behavior change. For example, binge-eating behavior may be followed by tension release (a positive consequence) and money spent (a negative consequence). For some people under certain conditions, the tension release is more meaningful and salient than the loss of money; hence, the tension release has greater reinforcement strength, and the binge-eating behavior tends to be maintained. In order to successfully change this behavior, patients need to become aware of and to evaluate the relative power that they ascribe to each consequence of the behavior.

Time: Immediate versus Delayed

These different consequences—positive or negative—follow the response network at different time intervals. For this reason, consequences are often classified along a temporal dimension. *Immediate* consequences are those that closely follow the response network. *Delayed* consequences are those that follow the response network after a period of time. The longer the consequences are delayed, the less influence they will have on the response network.

Patients need to become aware of *when* consequences follow their responses. As we noted earlier, most patients are unaware of the consequences to their behavior. When they do become aware of these consequences, they tend to be more cognizant of the immediate as opposed to the delayed ones. Hence, patients who have eating disorders tend to be more aware of the immediate consequences of their unhealthy eating habits (e.g., feeling satisfied, gaining emotional relief) and less aware of the delayed consequences (e.g., jeopardizing relationships, developing medical/dental problems). In fact, for many patients, the long-term consequences of their unhealthy eating habits often go unheeded.

Basic Formula for Making Changes in Eating Behavior

The basic formula for facilitating change involves helping patients to:

1. Identify the *cue* that triggers their responses.
2. Label their thoughts, feelings, and behaviors—that is, label their *responses.*
3. Identify the *consequences* and determine how each consequence influences patients' network of responses.

Patients are introduced to this model in sessions 2 and 3. The Eating Behaviors Self-Monitoring Worksheet (Form 1.2) is kept by patients throughout the program, starting with session 1. This worksheet helps patients and therapist identify binge-eating episodes along with their cues and consequences. As noted, patients who have eating disorders characteristically demonstrate (1) problems with control, (2) unhealthy eating habits, and (3) erroneous ideas and faulty assumptions about food, eating, body weight, and body shape. The Restructuring Thoughts Worksheet (Form 4.2) is used to help patients understand and master these three problem areas by:

1. Becoming aware of the automatic nature of their inappropriate or unhealthy responses.
2. Identifying the misconceptions and overvalued ideas that accompany their inappropriate feelings and behaviors.
3. Providing a framework for learning self-control strategies (e.g., restricting or changing the cue, building in self-rewards [positive consequences], deliberately selecting a pleasant and meaningful alternative response).

This worksheet differentiates automatic from deliberate and immediate versus delayed consequences (and positive vs. negative). These differentiations are useful for the therapist to understand and use but are not included in the materials provided to the patients.

The Need to Individualize Treatment

It is important to keep in mind that these treatment guidelines are intended to be just what they are—guidelines. They need to be tailored to fit the individual patient's needs, level of understanding, and pace. Be prepared to modify the probes as the session unfolds. Moreover, certain patients may need to learn cognitive restructuring in a stepwise fashion by mastering one step before proceeding to the next.

Practitioners interested in more detailed guidelines on the various thought restructuring (or cognitive restructuring) techniques—such as challenging faulty attributions, decatastrophizing, challenging all-or-none thinking, exploring alternatives, eliciting predictions, in addition to changing faulty notions and beliefs—are referred to other resources, such as those that close this section.

Additional Resources

Background reading in a variety of texts on BED and CBT may be of use for many clinicians. Articles and presentations reporting the results of the research on this manual are also included:

Agras, W. S. (Ed.). (1998). *Overcoming eating disorders: A cognitive-behavioral treatment for bulimia nervosa and binge-eating disorder: Therapist guide.* Orlando, FL: Psychological Corporation.

American Psychiatric Association. (2006). *Practice guidelines for the treatment of psychiatric disorders: Compendium 2006.* Arlington, VA: Author.

Brewerton, T. D. (Ed.). (2004). *Clinical handbook of eating disorders.* New York: Marcel Dekker.

Fairburn, C. G., & G. Wilson. (Eds.). (1993). *Binge eating: Nature, assessment, and treatment.* New York: Guilford Press.

Grilo, C. M. (Ed.). (2006). *Eating and weight disorders.* New York: Psychology Press.

Mitchell, J. E. (Ed.). (2001). *The outpatient treatment of eating disorders: A guide for therapists, dietitians, and physicians.* Minneapolis: University of Minnesota Press.

Munsch, S., & Beglinger, C. (Eds.). (2005). *Obesity and binge eating disorder.* New York: Karger.

Norring, C., & Palmer, R. L. (Eds.). (2005). *EDNOS, eating disorders not otherwise specified: Scientific and clinical perspectives on the other eating disorders.* London: Routledge.

Peterson, C. B., Mitchell, J. E., Crow, S. J., Crosby, R. D., & Wonderlich, S. A. (2006, August). *A randomized comparison trial of group treatment models for binge eating disorder.* Paper presented at the annual meeting of the Eating Disorders Research Society, Port Douglas, Australia.

Peterson, C. B., Mitchell, J. E., Engbloom, S., Nugent, S., Mussell M. P., Crow, S. J., et al. (2001). Self-help versus therapist-led group cognitive-behavioral treatment of binge eating disorder at follow-up. *International Journal of Eating Disorders, 30*(4), 363–374.

Peterson, C. B., Mitchell, J. E., Engbloom, S., Nugent, S., Mussell, M. P., & Miller, J. P. (1998). Group cognitive-behavioral treatment of binge eating disorder: A comparison of therapist-led vs. self-help formats. *International Journal of Eating Disorders, 24,* 125–136.

Schmidt, U., & Treasure, J. (Eds.). (1997). *Clinician's guide to getting better bit(e) by bit(e): A survival guide for sufferers of bulimia nervosa and binge eating disorders.* Hove, East Sussex, UK: Psychology Press.

Thompson, J. K. (Ed.). (2004). *Eating disorders and obesity.* Hoboken, NJ: Wiley.

Session-by-Session
Therapist Guidelines

SESSION I. Program Overview and What Is Binge-Eating Disorder?   85

SESSION 2. Cues and Consequences, Part I   87

SESSION 3. Cues and Consequences, Part II   89

SESSION 4. Thoughts, Feelings, and Behaviors   91

SESSION 5. Restructuring Your Thoughts   93

SESSION 6. Cues and Chains   94

SESSION 7. Impulsivity, Self-Control, and Mood Enhancement   96

SESSION 8. Body Image, Part I   98

SESSION 9. Body Image, Part II   99

SESSION 10. Self-Esteem   101

SESSION 11. Stress Management and Problem Solving   102

SESSION 12. Assertiveness   104

SESSION 13. Weight Management   105

SESSION 14. Relapse Prevention, Part I: Exposure to High-Risk Foods and Situations   106

SESSION 15. Relapse Prevention, Part II: Review of Progress and Long-Term Planning   108

Program Overview
and What Is Binge-Eating Disorder?

Session Content

Program overview
Making a commitment to change
What is binge-eating disorder?: Psychoeducation on binge-eating disorder
What to expect as you change your eating behavior
Assign homework for session 2

> Complete Eating Behaviors Self-Monitoring Worksheet daily (Form 1.2).
> Complete Reasons for and against Changing Unhealthy Eating Habits worksheet (Form 1.3).
> Complete Alternatives to Binge-Eating Worksheet (Form 1.4).
> Read Session 2 Lecture Handout (Form 2.1).

Materials Needed for This Session

Form 1.1. Session 1 Lecture Handout
Form 1.2. Eating Behaviors Self-Monitoring Worksheet
Form 1.3. Reasons for and against Changing Unhealthy Eating Habits worksheet
Form 1.4. Alternatives to Binge-Eating Worksheet
Form 2.1. Session 2 Lecture Handout

About Session 1

This session provides both an overview of the program, detailing the material to be covered, and psychoeducational information about binge-eating disorder. In this session, as in all sessions, an effort should be made to personalize the material whenever possible and, in particular, to ask patients to illustrate or give examples of points that are made in the reading materials.

The material covered in the section "What to Expect as You Change Your Eating Behavior" is particularly important. Many patients find that when they are struggling with trying to eliminate binge eating that they experience uncomfortable affects that have been suppressed by the binge eating. Their emotional lability may worsen somewhat before they are able to gain ongoing control of their eating behavior. Anticipating this fluctuation can be quite helpful for patients.

Homework

Three forms are assigned as homework for session 2. The first is Form 1.2, Eating Behaviors Self-Monitoring Worksheet. Patients complete this worksheet regularly throughout treatment. An example of how to fill out this form is shown in the upper-right-hand corner. Patients are asked to indicate meals or snacks with a box, to indicate binge-eating episodes with a line, and to make the length of the line reflect the duration of the binge-eating episode. They are also asked to start identifying cues, and it is useful to illustrate for them what sorts of cues many people frequently report. Examples on the sheet include anger and boredom—the latter being probably the single most common reason for binge eating cited by patients. It is important for patients to start to identify the precipitants or cues for their individual binge-eating episodes. It is also useful for patients to check whether or not they are menstruating because sometimes menstruation precipitates an exacerbation of binge-eating behavior, and also to indicate days in which they are successful in avoiding binge eating. In subsequent sessions, when this form is reviewed it is important to examine not only binge-eating behavior but also the pattern of meals and snacks. For example, if the patient indicates an eating episode at 8:00 A.M., which represents breakfast, it is important to talk about what constitutes breakfast. Many of these patients tend not to eat breakfast or to eat a very small breakfast and a very small lunch, anticipating that they will overeat later in the day. This pattern increases the likelihood that they will actually binge eat.

As with other homework assignments, patients are initially somewhat reticent to complete this form. Much emphasis needs to be placed on the importance of this form, and if necessary, time should be devoted during the session for its completion.

Patients are also asked to fill out Form 1.3, Reasons for and against Changing Unhealthy Eating Habits. Examples of the sort of items that subjects might insert are shown below.

Sample of Form 1.3

REASONS FOR AND AGAINST CHANGING
UNHEALTHY EATING HABITS WORKSHEET

In the left-hand column, list your reasons *for* stopping your unhealthy eating habits. In the right-hand column, list your reasons *against* stopping your unhealthy eating habits.

Reasons for Stopping   Reasons against Stopping

Feel in control   *Food comforts me*

Save money   *Will get angry*

Less depressed   *Hard to quit*

Patients are also asked to fill out Form 1.4, Alternatives to Binge-Eating Worksheet. A number of possible alternatives are already listed on the form, with blanks provided for patient additions.

Cues and Consequences, Part I

Session Content

Review homework
Session agenda

    Cues and consequences: definitions
    Categories of cues and consequences
        Social, situational, physiological–nutritional, mental
    Cues that trigger binge-eating behaviors
    Consequences of binge-eating behaviors: positive and negative
    Strategies for change
        Rearranging cues
        Changing response to cues
        Rearranging consequences

Assign homework for session 3

    Continue to complete Self-Monitoring Worksheet (Form 1.2).
    Complete Rearranging Cues Worksheet (Form 2.2).
    Complete Rearranging Consequences: Goal-Setting and Self-Rewards Worksheet (Form 2.3).
    Read Session 3 Lecture Handout (Form 3.1).

Materials Needed for This Session

Form 1.2.   Eating Behaviors Self-Monitoring Worksheet
Form 2.1   Session 2 Lecture Handout
Form 2.2   Rearranging Cues Worksheet, Part I: Changing Your Response
Form 2.3   Rearranging Consequences: Goal-Setting and Self-Rewards Worksheet
Form 3.1   Session 3 Lecture Handout

About Session 2

Session 2 involves an in-depth assessment of cues and consequences as well as an early examination of the response set, which includes thoughts, feelings, and behaviors. Emphasis in this session should be placed on pinning down specific cues that may be involved in the patient's binge eating, and specific consequences that may follow. Again, as the therapist goes through this material with the patient, it is important to elicit examples of specific cues and consequences encountered in relation to her or his eating behaviors. There is then a section on dealing with cues, and the homework section includes the usual Eating Behaviors Self-Monitoring Worksheet, instructions for Rearranging Cues . . . and Changing Your Response, as well as a section on Rearranging Consequences . . . and Goal Setting and Self-Rewards. An example of the type of material that might be included in Form 2.2 is shown.

Sample of Form 2.2

REARRANGING CUES WORKSHEET, PART I: CHANGING YOUR RESPONSE

Think of the three cues that are frequently associated with binge eating. Consider strategies that you can use to rearrange or change your response to the cue.

Cue   *Driving by the bakery* _____

Strategy *Take a different route home* _____

_____

_____

Cue   *The vending machine at work* _____

Strategy *Not have extra cash at work* _____

_____

_____

Cue   _____

Strategy _____

_____

_____

The rearranging consequences–self-reward section is straightforward and self-explanatory.

Cues and Consequences, Part II

Session Content

Review homework
Session agenda

Prolonged dieting and hunger cues may lead to binge eating
A vicious cycle: diet, binge-eat, feel guilty, attempt to diet, binge-eat again
Recommendations for healthy eating
Planning meals
Exercise and weight management

Assign homework for session 4

Continue to complete Eating Behaviors Self-Monitoring Worksheet (Form 1.2).
Complete Rearranging Cues Worksheet, Part II: Hunger and Chaotic Eating (Form 3.2).
Read and complete Healthy Exercise Worksheet (Form 3.3).
Read the Meal Plan Worksheet (Form 3.4) and try to plan your meals in the evening for the next day; do this for at least 3 days.
Select a goal for the week and a reward.

Materials Needed for This Session

Form 1.2.   Eating Behaviors Self-Monitoring Worksheet
Form 3.1.   Session 3 Lecture Handout
Form 3.2.   Rearranging Cues, Part II: Hunger and Chaotic Eating
Form 3.3.   Healthy Exercise Worksheet
Form 3.4.   Meal Plan Worksheet
Form 4.1.   Session 4 Lecture Handout

About Session 3

In session 3 strong emphasis is placed on the development of meal-planning behaviors and the establishment of a pattern of healthy exercise as well as additional work on rearranging cues. The homework assignment includes the Rearranging Cues worksheet (Form 3.2) and Healthy Exercise Worksheet (Form 3.3), which are self-explanatory. Patients are asked to fill out a Meal

Plan Worksheet (Form 3.4). For therapists who are less familiar with this aspect, a healthy example is shown below.

Sample of Form 3.4

MEAL PLAN WORKSHEET

Meal/snack	Time	Check when eaten
Breakfast *Cereal with 2% milk* *Piece of whole wheat toast with margarine*	7:30 AM	
Morning snack *Apple*	10 AM	
Lunch *Sandwich with turkey, cheese, lettuce,* *tomato, and mayo* *Small bowl of applesauce*	12 noon	
Afternoon snack *Crackers and cheese*	3 PM	
Dinner *Peas* *Baked potato* *Chicken* *Margarine*	6 PM	
Evening snack *Glass of 2% milk*	9 PM	

Thoughts, Feelings, and Behaviors

Session Content

Review homework
Session agenda

    The thought–behavior connection
    Automatic thoughts
    Problematic styles of thinking

Assign homework for session 5

    Continue to complete Eating Behaviors Self-Monitoring Worksheet (Form 1.2).
    Complete Restructuring Thoughts Worksheets (Form 4.2):
        Pick a cue that you have identified.
        Write down corresponding thoughts, feelings, behaviors, and consequences.
        Leave bottom half ("Revised Thoughts," etc.) blank for now; you will complete it after
            the next session.
    Read Session 5 Lecture Handout (Form 5.1).
    Select a goal for the week and a reward.

Materials Needed for This Session

Form 1.2.   Eating Behaviors Self-Monitoring Worksheet
Form 4.1.   Session 4 Lecture Handout
Form 4.2.   Restructuring Thoughts Worksheet
Form 5.1.   Session 5 Lecture Handout

About Session 4

Session 4 focuses on the response set as opposed to the cues and consequences. Because some patients have a great deal of difficulty sorting out thoughts versus feelings, it is important for the therapist to be able to label these appropriately so that the patient can begin to grasp the subtle differences. The Styles of Thinking section in Form 4.1 offers a categorization scheme, but this is less important than having subjects identify thinking styles that are dysfunctional for them, even if they don't necessarily fit into one of these categories. In terms of homework for session 5, patients need to start completing the Restructuring Thoughts Worksheets. It is useful to go over at least one worksheet with the patient prior to sending her or him home to complete the homework. An example is shown below.

CUE	RESPONSES		CONSEQUENCES
Get dressed. Pull on jeans.	THOUGHTS I'm fat! My jeans are too tight!	BEHAVIORS Not eat breakfast or lunch.	Very hungry. Binge-eat in evening when get home.
	FEELINGS Sadness Fear, anxiety		
	REVISED THOUGHTS My jeans shrunk. My jeans are too small for me—I'm older now.	REVISED BEHAVIORS Eat breakfast and lunch.	REVISED CONSEQUENCES Avoid binge-eating episode.
	REVISED FEELINGS Relief		

Restructuring Your Thoughts

Session Content

Review homework
Session agenda

    Evaluating your thoughts (Restructuring Step 2)
        Method 1: Challenge problem thoughts by questioning them
        Method 2: Challenge problem thoughts by testing them
    Change your thoughts (Restructuring Step 3)
    Determine the effects of your revised thoughts (Restructuring Step 4)

Assign homework for session 5

    Continue to complete Eating Behaviors Self-Monitoring Worksheets (Form 1.2).
    Complete Restructuring Thoughts Worksheet (Form 4.2).
    Read Session 6 Lecture Handout (Form 6.1).
    Select goal for week and reward.

Materials Needed for This Session

Form 1.2.   Eating Behaviors Self-Monitoring Worksheet
Form 4.2.   Restructuring Thoughts Worksheet
Form 6.1.   Session 6 Lecture Handout

About Session 5

Session 5 continues to focus on restructuring thoughts by offering different methods by which problematic thoughts can be challenged. The first is by directly questioning the evidence for the thoughts and the second involves prospective hypothesis testing of individual thoughts. The homework assignment includes the Restructuring Thoughts Worksheet plus the usual Self-Monitoring Worksheet.

Cues and Chains

Session Content

Review homework
Session agenda

Review cue–response–consequences sequence.
Explain how consequences become cues in a longer behavioral chain.
Use change strategies to interrupt the chain.

Assign homework for session 6

Continue to complete Eating Behaviors Self-Monitoring Worksheet (Form 1.2).
Complete the Identifying Behavioral Chains Worksheet (Form 6.2).
Read Session 7 Lecture Handout (Form 7.1).
Select goal for the week and a reward.

Materials Needed for This Session

Form 1.2.   Eating Behaviors Self-Monitoring Worksheet
Form 6.1.   Session 6 Lecture Handout
Form 6.2.   Identifying Behavioral Chains Worksheet
Form 7.1.   Session 7 Lecture Handout

About Session 6

Session 6 introduces the idea of cues and chains. It is important for patients to understand that this idea is a logical extension of the cue–response–consequence set. Basically, patients record their cues, responses, and consequences over the course of a period of time, often as long as a day, to see how certain consequences become cues for the next response set. This transition can be difficult for some patients, but most understand the idea of the chain fairly quickly. The homework for this session again focuses on the Self-Monitoring Worksheet as well as Identifying Behavioral Chains; several examples are included in the manual. It is important to demonstrate to patients how to interrupt chains by intervening at certain points. This process is illustrated below in the following figure.

Sample of Form 6.2

IDENTIFYING BEHAVIORAL CHAINS WORKSHEET

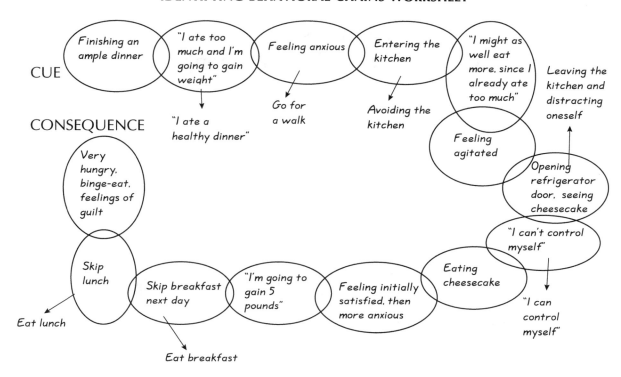

Impulsivity, Self-Control, and Mood Enhancement

Session Content

Review homework
Session agenda

    Managing your impulses
        Self-control can be learned
        Strategies for self-control
    Mood enhancement
        Pleasant events and your mood
        Increasing pleasant events

Assign homework for session 7

    Continue to complete Eating Behaviors Self-Monitoring Worksheet (Form 1.2).
    Complete Changing Impulsivity Worksheet (Form 7.2).
    Complete Pleasant Activities Worksheet (Form 7.3).
    Read Session 8 Lecture Handout (Form 8.1).
        Choose a strategy for managing impulses and practice it for the week.
        Select a reward for using an impulse control strategy.
        Plan to increase the number of pleasant activities you do this week; then keep track of the number of activities you do and rate your mood daily.

Materials Needed for This Session

Form 1.2.   Eating Behaviors Self-Monitoring Worksheet
Form 7.1.   Session 7 Lecture Handout
Form 7.2.   Changing Impulsivity Worksheet
Form 7.3.   Pleasant Activities Worksheet
Form 8.1.   Session 8 Lecture Handout

About Session 7

Session 7 focuses on three related areas: impulsivity, self-control, and mood enhancement. Most patients find this area fairly straightforward. The homework assignments should be illustrated before the patient leaves the session—for example, as the patient describes situations in which she or he tends to be impulsive (around food or not around food). Also, most patients can readily indicate a number of pleasant activities that they would like to pursue for mood enhancement.

SESSION 8

Body Image, Part I

Session Content

Review homework
Session agenda

What is body Image?
What influences body image?
   Family, peers, childhood, adult experiences, and culture
Body image and binge-eating disorder
Improving your body image

Assign homework for session 8

Continue to complete Eating Behaviors Self-Monitoring Worksheet (Form 1.2).
Complete Cultural and Family Influences on Body Image Worksheet (Form 8.2).
Complete Changing Your Thoughts about Your Body Worksheet (Form 8.3).
Read Session 9 Lecture Handout (Form 9.1).
Select a goal and reward for the week.

Materials Needed for This Session

Form 1.2. Eating Behaviors Self-Monitoring Worksheet
Form 8.1. Session 8 Lecture Handout
Form 8.2. Cultural and Family Influences on Body Image Worksheet
Form 8.3. Changing Your Thoughts about Your Body Worksheet
Form 9.1   Session 9 Lecture Handout

About Session 8

Many people are generally aware that cultural and family influences are important but have never actually stopped to "pin them down." It can be quite useful to have patients do so, and to initiate this process prior to their leaving the session. The materials to be completed are fairly straightforward.

SESSION 9

Body Image, Part II

Session Content

Review homework
Session agenda

> Changing your thinking about body image
> Affirmations
> Suggestions for improving body perception

Assign homework for session 9

> Continue to complete Eating Behaviors Self-Monitoring Worksheet (Form 1.2).]
> Complete Affirmations Worksheet (Form 9.2).
> Read Session 10 Lecture Handout (Form 10.1).
> Add to list of suggestions for Improving Body Perception.
> Select a goal and reward for the week.

Materials Needed for This Session

Form 1.2.   Eating Behaviors Self-Monitoring Worksheet
Form 9.1.   Session 9 Lecture Handout
Form 9.2.   Affirmations Worksheet
Form 10.1. Lecture Handout for Session 10

About Session 9

In this second body image lecture quite a bit of material is devoted to affirmations, which can be quite useful for patients. Examples of affirmations are shown below.

Sample of Form 9.2

AFFIRMATIONS WORKSHEET

How you think about and talk to yourself can improve your body image and your self-image.

List five positive statements about your body:

1. *I like my eyes.*
2. *My legs allow me to run.*
3. *I have a nice smile.*
4.
5.

Now list five positive statements about yourself that do not relate to your physical appearance (e.g., personality, sense of humor):

1. *People like my sense of humor.*
2. *People seem to like to be with me.*
3. *I am a good listener.*
4.
5.

If you have difficulty with either part of this exercise, try to think of how your friends and family might describe your positive qualities.

SESSION 10

Self-Esteem

Session Content

Review homework
Session agenda

    How do you define yourself?
    Testing the accuracy of negative self-evaluations
    The self-concept inventory
        More on revising weaknesses

Assign homework for session 10

    Continue to complete Eating Behaviors Self-Monitoring Worksheet (Form 1.2).
    Complete Self-Concept Inventory (Form 10.2).
    Read Session 11 Lecture Handout (Form 11.1).
    Select goals and rewards for each of the next 2 weeks.

Materials Needed for This Session

Form 1.2.   Eating Behaviors Self-Monitoring Worksheet
Form 10.1. Session 10 Lecture Handout
Form 10.2. Self-Concept Inventory
Form 11.1. Session 11 Lecture Handout

About Session 10

Session 10 focuses on self-concept and includes a Self-Concept Inventory. Again most patients can readily complete this form. It is important to stress that this inventory should cover both positive and negative attributes. A preview of behavioral problem solving, introduced in detail in session 11, may be useful here. Note that sessions are now spaced 2 weeks apart. The goal-and-reward component should cover the next 2 weeks until session 11.

SESSION 11

Stress Management and Problem Solving

Session Content

Review homework
Session agenda

    How do you deal with stress?
    What is stress?
        Stressors
        Stress responses
    How to manage stress
        Problem solving: Managing the stressor
        Stress management: Managing the stress response

Assign homework for session 11

    Continue to complete Eating Behaviors Self-Monitoring Worksheet (Form 1.2).
    Read Learning to Handle Mistakes (Form 11.2).
    Read Principles of Acceptance and Self-Acceptance (Form 11.3).
    Complete Stress Reduction Experiment Worksheet (Form 11.4).
    Read Session 12 Lecture Handout (Form 12.1).
    Select goals and rewards for the next 2 weeks.

Materials Needed for This Session

Form 1.2.   Eating Behaviors Self-Monitoring Worksheet
Form 11.1. Session 11 Lecture Handout
Form 11.2. Learning to Handle Mistakes
Form 11.3. Principles of Acceptance and Self Acceptance
Form 11.4. Stress Reduction Experiment Worksheet
Form 12.1. Session 12 Lecture Handout

About Session 11

Session 11 focuses on stress management and problem solving. Some of this material has been covered in other ways earlier in the manual. It is important, however, for patients to develop ways of examining specific stressors in their environment and appropriate stress management techniques. Again, most of this material is straightforward, but the ideas are usually not considered systematically by patients. Homework assignments include Learning to Handle Mistakes, Principles of Acceptance and Self-Acceptance, and the Stress Reduction Experiment Worksheet. Prior to ending the session, it may be useful to ask patients to identify a stressor they wish to consider to get them started.

SESSION 12

Assertiveness

Session Content

Review homework
Session agenda

> What is assertiveness?
> How self-talk can lead to passive, aggressive, or assertive behaviors
> Nonverbal behaviors
> Suggested assertive self-statements

Assign homework for session 12

> Continue to complete Eating Behaviors Self-Monitoring Worksheet (Form 1.2).
> Complete Thoughts Associated with Assertive and Nonassertive Behavior Worksheet (Form 12.2).
> Read Session 13 Lecture Handout (Form 13.1).
> Select goals and rewards for the next 2 weeks.

Materials Needed for This Session

Form 1.2.   Eating Behaviors Self-Monitoring Worksheet
Form 12.1. Session 12 Lecture Handout
Form 12.2. Thoughts Associated with Assertive and Nonassertive Behavior Worksheet
Form 13.1. Session 13 Lecture Handout

About Session 12

The material covered here is usually very accessible for most patients, although differentiating assertive from passive and aggressive behavior is sometimes surprising for patients, particularly those for whom passivity has been an ongoing problem. The homework for session 12 includes the Thoughts Associated with Assertive and Nonassertive Behavior Worksheet (Form 12.2).

SESSION 13

Weight Management

Session Content

Review homework
Session agenda

> What is a healthy weight for you?
> Strategies for maintaining a healthy weight
>> Healthy exercise
>> What you eat
> Don't put life on hold until you lose weight

Assign homework for session 13

> Continue to complete Eating Behaviors Self-Monitoring Worksheet (Form 1.2).
> Complete Activities You Are Putting Off until You Lose Weight Worksheet (Form 13.2).
> Complete High-Risk Foods and Situations Worksheet (Form 13.3).
> Read Session 14 Lecture Handout (Form 14.1).

Materials Needed for This Session

Form 1.2.   Eating Behaviors Self-Monitoring Worksheet
Form 13.1. Session 13 Lecture Handout
Form 13.2. Activities You Are Putting Off Until You Lose Weight Worksheet
Form 13.3. High-Risk Foods and Situations Worksheet
Form 14.1. Session 14 Lecture Handout

About Session 13

Session 13 returns to the issue of weight management by emphasizing weight maintenance. However, when working with a BED patient who clearly is overweight, you may discuss weight reduction techniques. There is no evidence that some dietary restriction will result in a worsening of binge eating, if done in a supportive context with eating guidelines that are flexible, not rigid. Given the health benefits of reductions in weight, this component needs to be considered for overweight or obese patients, particularly those with a BMI > 30. The issue of including some dietary restrictions will need to be handled on a patient-by-patient basis. It is important to help patients begin to work on high-risk foods and situations as well.

SESSION 14

Relapse Prevention, Part I
Exposure to High-Risk Foods and Situations

Session Content

Review homework
Session agenda

    Planning to prevent relapse
    How to practice exposure to high-risk foods and situations
    Tips for successful exposures
    Questions to help your relapse prevention planning

Assign homework for session 14

    Continue to complete Eating Behaviors Self-Monitoring Worksheet (Form 1.2).
    Complete Relapse Scenario Worksheet (Form 14.2) also using a Restructuring Thoughts
        Worksheet (Form 4.2).
    Complete Lapse Plan and Relapse Plan Worksheet (Form 14.3).
    Complete Exposures for High-Risk Foods Worksheet (Form 14.4).
    Complete Exposures for High-Risk Situations Worksheet (Form 14.5).
    Read Session 15 Lecture Handout (Form 15.1).

Materials Needed for This Session

Form 1.2.   Eating Behaviors Self-Monitoring Worksheet
Form 4.2.   Restructuring Thoughts Worksheet
Form 14.1. Session 14 Lecture Handout
Form 14.2. Relapse Scenario Worksheet
Form 14.3. Lapse Plan and Relapse Plan Worksheet
Form 14.4. Exposures for High-Risk Foods Worksheet
Form 14.5. Exposures for High-Risk Situations Worksheet
Form 15.1. Session 15 Lecture Handout

About Session 14

The last two sessions, 14 and 15, deal with relapse prevention. Most patients have reduced or eliminated their binge-eating behavior at this point in treatment. The emphasis now is on maintaining the changes over time. In this session, focus on differentiating lapses (temporary setbacks) from relapses (wherein the person returns to her or his previous pattern of behavior on an ongoing basis). Lapses should be regarded as opportunities to learn and in no way indicative of a negative outcome. In contrast, relapses should be avoided. This is a particularly difficult time for patients and having them actually discuss lapse versus relapse in some detail may be helpful.

These sessions also include detailed planning on to how to engage in purposeful exposures to high-risk foods and situations. It is important for patients to not live in fear that they will relapse if they encounter certain foods or situations, because such occasions will likely arise.

Relapse Prevention, Part II
Review of Progress and Long-Term Planning

Session Content

Review homework
Session agenda

    Recognize your progress; praise your accomplishments
    Keep practicing the skills you've learned
    Plan a health lifestyle

Materials Needed for This Session

Form 15.1. Session 15 Lecture Handout
Form 15.2. Recognize Your Progress
Form 15.3. Health Lifestyle Plan

About Session 15

This is the final session of the program. Help patients recognize and acknowledge the progress they have made over the course of the treatment. Patients should leave the program on a positive note. Briefly review the skills and strategies covered in the program and encourage their continued use. Ask patients to continue to use the manual, reviewing the sessions they found particularly useful.

Patient Materials

Session-by-Session Lecture Handouts and Worksheets

FORM 1.1.   Session 1 Lecture Handout   111

FORM 1.2.   Eating Behaviors Self-Monitoring Worksheet   115

FORM 1.3.   Reasons for and against Changing Unhealthy Eating Habits Worksheet   116

FORM 1.4.   Alternatives to Binge-Eating Worksheet   117

FORM 2.1.   Session 2 Lecture Handout   118

FORM 2.2.   Rearranging Cues Worksheet, Part I: Changing Your Response   122

FORM 2.3.   Rearranging Consequences: Goal Setting and Self-Rewards Worksheet   123

FORM 3.1.   Session 3 Lecture Handout   124

FORM 3.2.   Rearranging Cues Worksheet, Part II: Hunger and Chaotic Eating   127

FORM 3.3.   Healthy Exercise Worksheet   128

FORM 3.4.   Meal Plan Worksheet   129

FORM 4.1.   Session 4 Lecture Handout   130

FORM 4.2.   Restructuring Thoughts Worksheet   134

FORM 5.1.   Session 5 Lecture Handout   135

FORM 6.1.   Session 6 Lecture Handout   138

FORM 6.2.   Identifying Behavioral Chains Worksheet   141

FORM 7.1.   Session 7 Lecture Handout   142

FORM 7.2.   Changing Impulsivity Worksheet   145

FORM 7.3.   Pleasant Activities Worksheet   146

FORM 8.1.   Session 8 Lecture Handout   147

FORM 8.2.   Cultural and Family Influences on Body Image Worksheet   150

FORM 8.3.   Changing Your Thoughts about Your Body Worksheet   151

FORM 9.1.   Session 9 Lecture Handout   152

FORM 9.2.   Affirmations Worksheet   154

FORM 10.1.   Session 10 Lecture Handout   155

FORM 10.2.   Self-Concept Inventory   158

FORM 11.1.   Session 11 Lecture Handout   160

FORM 11.2.   Learning to Handle Mistakes   165

FORM 11.3.   Principles of Acceptance and Self-Acceptance   166

FORM 11.4.   Stress Reduction Experiment Worksheet   167

FORM 12.1.   Session 12 Lecture Handout   168

FORM 12.2.   Thoughts Associated with Assertive and Nonassertive Behavior Worksheet   171

FORM 13.1.   Session 13 Lecture Handout   172

FORM 13.2.   Activities You Are Putting Off until You Lose Weight Worksheet   174

FORM 13.3.   High-Risk Foods and Situations Worksheet   175

FORM 14.1.   Session 14 Lecture Handout   176

FORM 14.2.   Relapse Scenario Worksheet   179

FORM 14.3.   Lapse Plan and Relapse Plan Worksheet   180

FORM 14.4.   Exposures for High-Risk Foods Worksheet   181

FORM 14.5.   Exposures for High-Risk Situations Worksheet   183

FORM 15.1.   Session 15 Lecture Handout   185

FORM 15.2.   Recognize Your Progress   187

FORM 15.3.   Healthy Lifestyle Plan   188

SESSION 1 LECTURE HANDOUT

Session 1. Overview/What Is Binge-Eating Disorder?

OVERVIEW OF THIS TREATMENT PROGRAM

This treatment is a structured program that uses psychoeducational and cognitive-behavioral techniques. The goals of the program are to help you:

- Interrupt binge eating.
- Establish healthy eating patterns.
- Identify and change problematic thoughts (self-talk) and negative feelings.
- Identify and use more effective coping strategies.

The basic program consists of 15 sessions and extends over a 20-week period: weekly for 10 weeks, then biweekly for 10 weeks. There are three phases. Phase I (sessions 1–6) emphasizes behavioral and cognitive strategies to target binge eating. Phase II (sessions 7–14) addresses associated problems that often accompany binge-eating behaviors. Phase III (sessions 14 and 15) focuses on maintaining improvement and preventing relapse.

Cognitive-behavioral therapy (CBT) was originally developed for the treatment of depression but has been used more recently to address eating problems, including binge eating. This type of treatment focuses on making changes in the "here-and-now" by using specific strategies to target factors that contribute to and maintain binge eating. CBT also addresses problematic thought patterns (self-talk) that have negative effects on behaviors and feelings.

Your Responsibilities

Attendance at all sessions is necessary. If you are unable to attend, please call and leave a message for your therapist indicating the reason for your absence.

If you experience difficulty with persistent suicidal thoughts, self-damaging behaviors such as cutting or other types of self-injury, or misuse of alcohol or other drugs, please tell a staff member immediately. More appropriate treatment will be recommended.

Making a Commitment to Change

Binge eating is a difficult problem to overcome for several reasons:

1. The habitual binge-eating cycle is similar to that of dependence on drugs or alcohol, but, unlike in chemical dependency treatment in which drug and alcohol are typically discontinued completely, one cannot stop eating.
2. Binge-eating behavior may reduce unpleasant feelings; many people find that binge eating is relaxing, stress reducing, or reinforcing in some way.
3. The feelings and behaviors associated with binge eating are perpetuated by problematic thoughts and misconceptions about food and weight.

4. Many people who binge-eat have had previous failures in treatment or on their own and fear having another failure; this program is designed to optimize the successful elimination of binge eating.

5. When binge-eating lessens or stops, individuals sometimes experience emotional ups and downs and other unpleasant symptoms; without a clear understanding of such symptoms, stopping the binge-eating behavior may be exceedingly difficult.

However, there are reasons to be hopeful. Many people have successfully stopped binge eating as a result of this program. The model used in this approach is a form of CBT that has now been used in two randomized trials, one conducted at the University of Minnesota and the second conducted at the University of Minnesota as well as at the Neuropsychiatric Research Institute in Fargo, North Dakota. The program is also quite similar to a number of other CBT programs that have been developed at other centers for treatment of individuals with BED. In these studies most patients benefit substantially; that is, they successfully learned to control their binge-eating behavior.

Recovery takes a lot of hard work and needs to be your *top priority*. You increase your chances of success if you make your treatment the #1 priority in your life right now.

The reading assignments, homework, and therapy sessions are designed to help you gain control over your eating behavior. Set aside time each day to read the manual and work on the assignments.

Development of Support

Individuals who binge-eat often report being socially isolated and feeling emotionally cut off from family, friends, and coworkers. The isolation may be due, in part, to the secretive nature of binge eating: spending a lot of time alone, hiding eating problems from others, and feeling ashamed about one's eating behaviors.

An important part of recovery is establishing and maintaining a healthy support system and learning specific ways to take care of yourself physically, emotionally, and spiritually.

Weight Management

This treatment is specifically designed to help you stop binge eating. Research has shown that individuals who are able to stop binge eating using this approach are less likely to gain weight in the future and may lose a small amount of weight after treatment. However, most people do not lose a significant amount of weight by eliminating binge eating. If you want to lose weight, stopping binge eating is an important first step. You may want to pursue additional weight loss strategies after you complete this treatment.

WHAT IS BINGE-EATING DISORDER?

Binge-eating disorder has the following characteristics:

- Binge eating occurs in 20–40% of people who are overweight.
- It occurs in 1–4% of the general population.
- It affects more women than men.
- It usually begins in late adolescence or early adulthood.
- People with the disorder have a history of dieting to lose weight.

Eating binges have these features:

- Rapid consumption of a large amount of food in a discrete period of time.
- A feeling of lack of control over eating behavior during binges.
- Feelings of remorse, distress, and guilt.

There are three kinds of negative consequences associated with binge eating:

1. Negative cognitive and emotional consequences, which can include:
   - Depression, anxiety
   - Irritability
   - Concentration problems
   - Self-criticism
2. Negative social and professional consequences, which can include:
   - Financial: loss of savings, debt
   - Isolation from family and friends
   - Work and school: decreased productivity, poor attendance
3. Negative physical consequences, which can include:
   - Weight gain: health risks

Important social, cultural, psychological, and physiological factors contribute to binge-eating disorder:

1. Factors in society and culture
   - Preoccupation with thinness and stigma against obesity
   - Emphasis on "youth"
   - Pressures to succeed, including weight control
2. Psychological factors
   - Body image disturbance: body dissatisfaction, overvaluing shape and weight
   - Low sense of self-worth and self-esteem
   - Low ability to cope with stressful situations
   - Impulsivity
3. Physiological–nutritional factors
   - Food deprivation—excess dieting, avoiding specific types of food
   - Heritability—weight range that is genetically determined

WHAT TO EXPECT AS YOU CHANGE YOUR EATING BEHAVIOR

The following sections include a brief description of changes that you may experience as you change your eating behavior. For some people, these changes will be very mild; for others, they will be more troublesome. If any of these changes are a problem for you, it is important that you talk about them during your sessions.

Changes in Thoughts and Feelings

For many people, binge eating serves to "stuff" or numb unpleasant or uncomfortable thoughts and feelings. When the binge eating stops, so do the anesthetic effects of the bingeing behavior.

As a result, you will probably become more aware of these unpleasant thoughts and feelings. Common changes to expect include becoming increasingly more aware of emotional pain, anger, loss, sadness, anxiety, or confusion. (The feeling of confusion is often associated with being unclear about what you want for yourself and how you are feeling.)

These unpleasant thoughts and feelings will decrease as you learn healthy responses to replace them.

Questioning, Uncertainty, and Anxiety

Whenever you are faced with something new, you can expect to experience some anxiety and to question the outcome. This stance is especially true when you are learning a new behavior and the outcome is uncertain—that is, when you have never experienced the outcome or you are unsure of the outcome.

One way to help you overcome anxiety and uncertainty is to remind yourself of the reasons for learning these new skills. These reasons include:

1. Being able to control many of the cues that trigger your unhealthy eating habits.
2. Having a flexible framework for controlling your eating behavior and maintaining a healthy weight.

HOMEWORK

1. Complete the Eating Behaviors Self-Monitoring Worksheet (Form 1.2) every day.
2. Complete Reasons for and against Changing Unhealthy Eating Habits Worksheet (Form 1.3).
3. Complete Alternatives to Binge Eating Worksheet (Form 1.4).
4. Read Session 2 Lecture Handout (Form 2.1).

Form 1.2

EATING BEHAVIORS SELF-MONITORING WORKSHEET

Name

INSTRUCTIONS:
1. Draw a line for each bingeing episode.
2. Make a box around the line for meals and snacks.
3. Please try to fill out this form each day.
4. Check **M** box at the end of the line when menstruating.
5. Check **A** box at the end of the line for abstinent days.
6. Indicate a cue, if a certain cue seemed to set off the binge-eating episode.

Example:

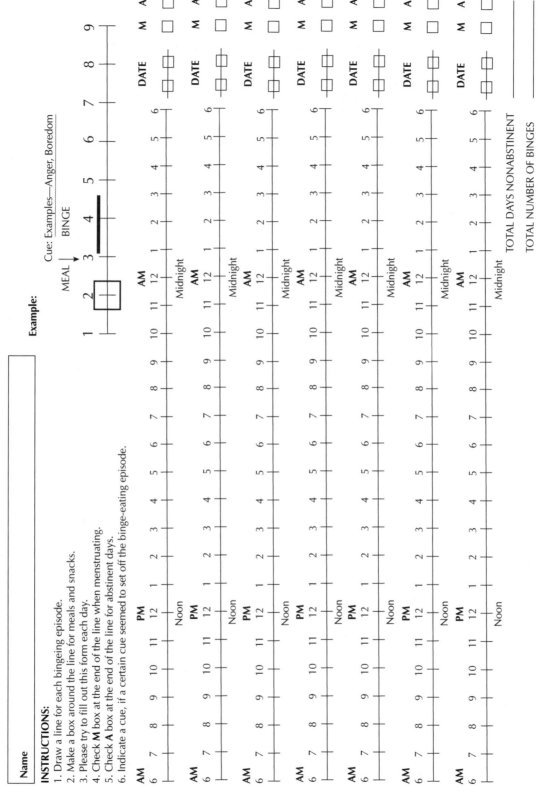

TOTAL DAYS NONABSTINENT

TOTAL NUMBER OF BINGES

115

From *Binge-Eating Disorder: Clinical Foundations and Treatment* by James E. Mitchell, Michael J. Devlin, Martina de Zwaan, Scott J. Crow, and Carol B. Peterson. Copyright 2008 by The Guilford Press. Permission to photocopy this form is granted to purchasers of this book for personal use only (see copyright page for details).

Form 1.3

REASONS FOR AND AGAINST CHANGING
UNHEALTHY EATING HABITS WORKSHEET

In the left-hand column, list your reasons *for* stopping your unhealthy eating habits.
In the right-hand column, list your reasons *against* stopping your unhealthy eating habits.

Reasons for Stopping   Reasons against Stopping

Form 1.4

ALTERNATIVES TO BINGE-EATING WORKSHEET

One of the most powerful ways of stopping binge eating is to engage in an alternative behavior when you are at risk of binge eating or when you have urges to binge eat. Circle the activities listed below that might work for you and list additional activities that may be useful alternatives for you:

1. Call a friend. Keep calling until you reach someone.

2. Take a bath or shower.

3. Take a walk.

4. Do a non-food-related activity outside the kitchen. Stay out of the kitchen.

5. Go to the library.

6. Do a relaxation exercise or meditation.

7. Distract yourself with a craft project, book, or TV program.

8. Read something inspirational.

9. Go to a movie, play, museum, etc.

10. Listen to music.

11. Clean or organize a room.

12. _____

13. _____

14. _____

SESSION 2 LECTURE HANDOUT

Session 2. Cues and Consequences, Part I

Our responses are cued by what happens before them. The word **CUE** refers to events that occur before responses (thoughts, feelings, or behaviors). Cues are also called "triggers" or "stimuli." They become associated with responses—in this case, binge eating.

Our responses are encouraged or discouraged by their results—that is, by those things that occur after the responses. The word **CONSEQUENCES** refers to events occurring after responses. Consequences can be positive and rewarding, which will make the response more likely to recur, or they can be negative, which will make the response less likely to recur. For the time being, think of responses as **BINGE-EATING BEHAVIORS.**

Cues and consequences can be grouped into the categories shown in the following figure.

Cues and consequences of binge-eating behaviors.

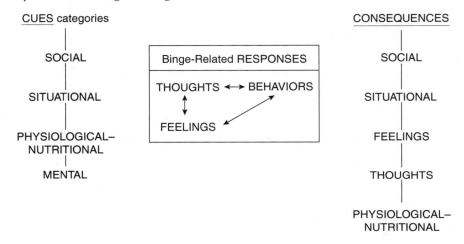

POSSIBLE *CUES* THAT TRIGGER BINGE-EATING BEHAVIORS

Categories	*Cues*
Social	1. Social isolation (boredom and loneliness)
	2. Interpersonal conflict (anger, frustration, self-blame)
	3. Social holidays and celebrations
	4. Observing others eat excessively
Situational	1. Advertisements in magazines, on TV, radio, or billboards
	2. Passing by a bakery or fast-food restaurant
	3. Eating "forbidden" or "fattening" foods
	4. Cooking dinner

Physiological–nutritional

    1. Hunger
    2. Fatigue

Mental

    1. Memory
    2. Mental image

POSSIBLE *CONSEQUENCES* THAT RESULT FROM BINGE-EATING BEHAVIORS

Consequences can be similarly separated into categories. Your unhealthy eating responses result in some positive consequences or they would not be maintained. They also result in negative consequences or there would be no need to change them. It is helpful to specify these differences, as follows:

Categories	*Positive Consequences*	*Negative Consequences*
Social	1. Avoiding interpersonal conflict or rejection	1. Social withdrawal 2. Lying and lack of trust in relationships 3. Problems from being overweight
Situational	1. Distraction from boring or unpleasant tasks 2. Avoiding responsibility	1. Occupational problems, procrastination 2. Financial problems
Feelings	1. Relief from tension, stress, anger 2. Relief from boredom 3. Emotional numbing 4. Feeling comfort or pleasure	1. Depression, guilt, shame, irritability, mood swings
Thoughts	1. Distraction from uncomfortable thoughts	1. Increase in negative self-esteem or guilt-related thoughts
Physiological–Nutritional	1. Reduction of hunger	1. Weight gain

The binge eating is maintained because the positive consequences resulting from binge-eating behaviors are more immediate than the negative consequences.

STRATEGIES FOR CHANGE: FOCUSING ON THE CUE

A major goal of treatment is to change your unhealthy eating habits. One way to change these habits is to take control of the cues by breaking up the relationship between the cues and your binge-eating responses. This is done by (1) rearranging cues and (2) changing your responses to cues. Some methods for breaking up the cue-to-response relationship are listed below.

Rearranging Cues

1. **Avoidance**—The simplest method of rearranging cues is to avoid the cue entirely. If a particular cue is a potent trigger for binge-eating behaviors, you can change your environment to remove the cue (e.g., don't walk by the bakery on the way to work; don't have hard candy available at home).
2. **Restricted Stimulus Field**—If you wish to reduce the frequency of problem behavior, restrict the cues that trigger that behavior (e.g., eat only at the table, away from other cues such as TV commercials; eat in the same place each time).
3. **Strengthen Cues for Desired Behavior**—Expose yourself to existing cues that lead more frequently to healthy behavior (e.g., study in the library if studying at home is associated with binge eating; eat meals with others if doing so prevents binge eating). Also, strengthen new cues by consistently associating them with responses that result in healthy consequences.

Changing Your Response to Cues

1. **Build in a Pause, Delay the Response**—Building in a pause allows time to pass and separates the cue from the automatic behavioral response (e.g., eating a candy bar is often a cue to binge-eat; create a pause of 15 minutes after eating the candy bar). Try to introduce increasingly longer pauses between the cue and binge eating. Often, the urge to binge-eat weakens with time.
2. **Alternative Behaviors**—Replace a problematic behavior with a healthier behavior that is adaptive. This method allows a more adaptive behavior to be associated with the high-risk cue (e.g., when a stressor triggers a desire to eat, go for a walk or call someone).
3. **Structure Your Environment for Response Prevention**— Structure your environment so that binge eating is unlikely or impossible following exposure to a cue (e.g., bring no money to work so you can't buy candy from the snack machine; eat with family or friends and take a walk afterward).

STRATEGIES FOR CHANGE: FOCUSING ON CONSEQUENCES

Another goal of treatment is to rearrange consequences of behavior so that appropriate behaviors are rewarded, whereas inappropriate behaviors are not. Rewarding yourself for not binge-eating can be a helpful strategy.

Rearranging Consequences

Guidelines for the use of rewards include the following:

1. The reward must follow rather than precede the behavior.
2. The reward must be contingent on the occurrence of the behavior (no behavior, no reward).
3. The reward should follow the behavior as quickly as possible.
4. Reward behavior in small steps (e.g., start with a reward for 1 hour free of binge eating, then 2 hours free, and so on).

Providing Rewards

There are two types of rewards: *mental* and *material or activity.*

Mental Rewards

It is important to congratulate yourself when you are making progress toward your goal. Tell yourself that you are succeeding, that you are doing a good job. Be sure to do this whenever you score even a minor victory. Telling yourself that you are making progress (when you are) can help you continue your gradual success.

Mental rewards are things that you imagine or say to yourself. They can include:

1. Complimenting yourself for something you have done.
2. Acknowledging characteristics of yourself that you value.
3. Imagining something pleasant.

In other words, mental rewards involve saying something positive to yourself about yourself or thinking about something pleasant.

Mental rewards are useful because:

1. They can be used anytime, anywhere.
2. They can be tailor-made (they come directly from you).
3. They can be given immediately after you accomplish a goal.

Material or Activity Rewards

Treat yourself to something fun or pleasurable (and easily obtainable) when you have accomplished your goal. Select rewards for reaching short-term (e.g., no binge eating for 1 day) and longer-term (e.g., no binge eating for 1 week) goals.

HOMEWORK

1. Continue to complete the Eating Behaviors Self-Monitoring Worksheet (Form 1.2).
2. Complete Rearranging Cues Worksheet, Part I: Changing Your Response (Form 2.2).
3. Complete Rearranging Consequences: Goal Setting and Self-Rewards Worksheet (Form 2.3).
4. Read Session 3 Lecture Handout (Form 3.1).

Form 2.2

REARRANGING CUES WORKSHEET, PART I:
CHANGING YOUR RESPONSE

Think of three cues that you frequently associate with binge eating. Consider strategies that you can use to rearrange or change your response to the cue.

Cue: _____

Strategy: _____

_____

_____

Cue: _____

Strategy: _____

_____

_____

Cue: _____

Strategy: _____

_____

_____

REARRANGING CONSEQUENCES:
GOAL SETTING AND SELF-REWARDS WORKSHEET

Self-rewards are an excellent way to encourage healthy behaviors. Setting up an effective reward system involves the following steps:

1. Define the goal behavior that you would like to achieve. Be specific in describing this goal behavior. Also, it is important to specify when and how frequently you want to accomplish this goal.

   Example: My goal behavior is to go for a walk after dinner each night.

   _____

   _____

   _____

   _____

   _____

2. Specify the reward for meeting your goal.

   Example: If I meet my goal, then I will take a bubble bath.

   _____

   _____

   _____

   _____

   _____

We encourage you to set weekly goals with rewards. Be sure to set realistic goals and to reward yourself immediately after reaching them.

SESSION 3 LECTURE HANDOUT

Session 3. Cues and Consequences, Part II

HUNGER AS A CUE: HOW TO NORMALIZE EATING BEHAVIORS

Many individuals with binge-eating disorder identify hunger as a frequent cue of binge-eating episodes. One of the causes of extreme hunger is severe dietary restriction. Many people report that the onset of their binge-eating behavior occurred following a prolonged period of dieting. In addition, many people find that their binge eating is triggered by dieting on an ongoing basis.

Research conducted in the late 1940s has helped us understand the nature of binge eating following food restriction. Dr. Ancel Keys conducted a study at the University of Minnesota in which healthy adult men (with no history of eating problems) were placed on a prolonged calorie-restricted diet. As a result of this semistarvation diet, these men became preoccupied with food. They also became depressed, anxious, and irritable, lost interest and pleasure in activities, tended to feel cold, and had trouble concentrating. When allowed to eat normally again, some men had binge-eating episodes. In addition, some gained weight above their original predieting weight. Eventually, the men stopped binge eating, returned to eating normally, and returned to their previous body weight.

Based on this study, it has been hypothesized that binge eating is a "natural" response to starvation and may have evolved in humans as a form of self-protection. For instance, if an animal in the wilderness experiences a shortage of food, it is adaptive for the animal to overeat when food then becomes available in order to "store up" energy for the next food shortage. Although this adaptation to starvation is considered unnecessary in our modern Western society (in which food tends to be abundant), the tendency to binge-eat in response to starvation or semistarvation was probably a biological necessity in the past and served to "protect" the human species.

The Keys study suggests that prolonged dieting may "trick" the body into believing that there is a shortage of food, resulting in a tendency to binge-eat at a later time. There is also some evidence that dieting may slow down an individual's metabolism, making her or him more prone to regain weight (although this effect is usually transient).

Another set of studies indicates that there are psychological risks of dieting as well. Research has found that when individuals deprive themselves of food and label foods "good" or "bad," they are more likely to overeat "forbidden" foods when they are eventually exposed to them. Viewing certain foods as "bad" and attempting to restrict them completely may lead to overeating.

People with binge-eating disorder often describe a vicious cycle in which they diet, binge-eat, feel guilty, attempt to diet, and end up binge eating again. People with binge-eating problems also describe a tendency toward chaotic eating patterns, which makes binge eating harder to stop. An important component of recovering from binge eating is to normalize your food intake and avoid excessive dieting.

RECOMMENDATIONS FOR HEALTHY EATING

1. Break the binge-eating–fasting cycle. We recommend eating three meals and two or three snacks each day to prevent the occurrence of extreme hunger. Often, it is helpful to focus on consuming regular meals and snacks first, then to focus on modifying their content.

2. Include all types of foods in your diet. Although we recommend following the "food pyramid" model to determine types and amounts of healthy food, it is important to avoid "forbidding" yourself to eat certain foods. In our view, all foods can be eaten in moderation. However, early in treatment when you first stop binge eating, you may find it helpful to avoid certain foods (e.g., sweets and high-fat foods) that tend to trigger your overeating episodes. You can reintroduce these foods later in treatment when your binge eating has improved.

3. Experiment with meal planning. Often, individuals with binge-eating disorder end up overeating when they decide what to eat on the spur of the moment. For this reason, planning the times and contents of your meals and snacks can be helpful in establishing normal eating patterns. Most people prefer to write out food plans for the following day on the preceding night. Others prefer to plan meals and snacks for the entire week. In addition to limiting on-the-spot decision making, writing down your food plans helps you prepare in advance for high-risk times. Many participants find it helpful to write food plans on the back of their Self-Monitoring Worksheets.

4. Many people fear that they will gain weight if they eat regular meals. Although you may experience some weight fluctuations when you first start to eat normally, most people with binge-eating disorder do not gain weight as a result of treatment. By reducing the frequency of binge-eating episodes as well as maintaining a healthy metabolism, regular food consumption does not usually lead to weight gain.

If weight loss is a goal for you, you can also start to change the content of the foods you eat. Exercise is a critical component, as is modifying your energy intake. One of the most effective strategies is to reduce (but not eliminate) your intake of high-fat foods. Try to substitute healthier, lower-fat alternatives. It helps to make sure that you have access to healthier food choices at home and at work. Setting small goals is helpful: For example, start by substituting a low-fat alternative once a day.

EXERCISE AND WEIGHT MANAGEMENT

One of the most important components of long-term weight management and health is regular exercise. It is important that you start to increase your activity level. Most people find that introducing exercise gradually is the most effective way to make it a long-term habit. For example, start by making small lifestyle changes: Take the stairs for one floor rather than the elevator; select a parking place further from the entrance; walk around the block after dinner. As you become more comfortable with an increased activity level, start to walk longer distances. Make sure to check with your doctor before you start exercising, especially if you have health concerns.

As you start to exercise, pay attention to what makes it more enjoyable for you. Do you prefer to exercise alone or with other people? What clothes are most comfortable for exercising? What time of day seems to work best? What activities do you enjoy? Determining these factors will increase the likelihood that you will continue to exercise. Also, make sure to set small goals and to reward yourself, especially at first.

Remember these steps for setting goals and selecting rewards:

1. **Setting goals:**
   - No goal is too small.
   - Don't choose too large a goal because you may set yourself up for failure.
   - You can always change your goals to make them more realistic and attainable.
2. **Selecting rewards for reaching your goals:**
   - Rewards should be things that make you feel good and are available (within your control).
   - Rewards should be powerful.
   - Rewards work best when they are immediately available.
   - Identify a menu of 10 rewards of different strengths.

HOMEWORK

1. Continue to complete the Eating Behaviors Self-Monitoring Worksheet (Form 1.2).
2. Complete Rearranging Cues Worksheet, Part II: Hunger and Chaotic Eating (Form 3.2).
3. Read and complete Healthy Exercise Worksheet (Form 3.3).
4. Read Meal Plan Worksheet (Form 3.4) and plan your meals on preceding evenings for at least 3 days.
5. Read Session 4 Lecture Handout (Form 4.1).
6. Set a goal for the week and a reward

Goal: _____

Reward: _____

Form 3.2

REARRANGING CUES WORKSHEET, PART II: HUNGER AND CHAOTIC EATING

Identify three cues related to hunger or chaotic eating that are associated with your binge-eating episodes. Consider strategies that you can use to rearrange or alter these cues.

Cue: _____

Strategy: _____

_____

_____

Cue: _____

Strategy: _____

_____

_____

Cue: _____

Strategy: _____

_____

_____

HEALTHY EXERCISE WORKSHEET

BENEFITS OF REGULAR EXERCISE

1. *Reduction of Stress*
   People who have used binge eating as a way to reduce stress and to relax often find it very helpful to exercise on a regular basis.

2. *Elevation of Mood*
   Regular exercise often improves mood and can help reduce and prevent negative feelings, including depression, anxiety, and irritability.

3. *Reaffirmation of Your Commitment to a Healthy Lifestyle*
   Regular exercise can contribute to an overall sense of well-being as well as provide a sense of success and accomplishment. Even small amounts of exercise can improve your health.

4. *Regulation of Metabolism and Weight*
   An individual's metabolic rate may be slowed by a period of food deprivation and dieting. Exercise can be useful in returning metabolic rate to normal and in maintaining long-term weight management.

5. *Opportunity to Socialize*

6. What additional benefits do you think regular exercise may have for you?

   _____

   _____

   _____

   _____

7. What steps can you take to increase your activity and to start to exercise?

   _____

   _____

   _____

Form 3.4

MEAL PLAN WORKSHEET

Meal/snack	Time	Check when eaten
Breakfast		
Morning snack		
Lunch		
Afternoon snack		
Dinner		
Evening snack		

Form 4.1

SESSION 4 LECTURE HANDOUT

Session 4. Thoughts, Feelings, and Behaviors

In the previous lectures, we discussed how specific cues trigger responses that lead to specific consequences. Cues trigger three types of responses: behaviors, thoughts, and feelings (see the following figure). Behaviors are external responses—actions that can be observed by others. Thoughts and feelings are internal responses. They are usually private and can be difficult for you to identify and for others to observe. Thoughts are particularly important in determining how a person reacts to a situation or cue.

Cues trigger three types of responses.

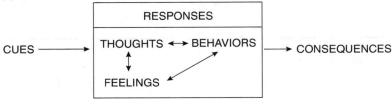

THE THOUGHT–BEHAVIOR CONNECTION

You may have observed that different people may react to the same situation in different ways. Reactions differ when peoples' thoughts (or "self-talk") about the situation are different. For example, two people pass a bakery after a stressful day at work. One person struggles with overeating. The other person does not have an eating problem. These two people may have very different reactions to seeing the bakery. The person with no eating problem may pay no attention to the bakery or maybe stop to buy bread or an after-dinner dessert. The person who struggles with binge eating may experience cravings and urges to binge-eat. He or she may begin buying binge foods for the evening. The two people have reacted differently to the same situation or cue.

The difference in their reactions is related to the difference in their thoughts about the bakery. The person with no eating problem may have thought, "It would be nice to have bread or dessert for dinner." The other person may have had one or more of these thoughts: "I haven't had anything to eat all day—I deserve something sweet"; "I need to binge-eat after a hard day"; "Nothing will help me relax except a binge"; or "I have to binge to get through the night."

There are a number of thoughts regarding your body, food, and yourself that are associated with problematic eating behaviors. Examples of these thoughts are:

"I'll get fat if I eat these cookies."

"I need to diet."

"I've eaten one bite, so I might as well eat the whole thing."

STARTING TO IDENTIFY AUTOMATIC THOUGHTS

You may not always be aware of your thoughts in response to situations. In fact, most people think automatically in response to situations or cues. For example, have you sometimes driven a car and couldn't remember how you got from one place to another? Obviously you were thinking, otherwise you could not have reached your destination, but you were not aware of the behaviors and thoughts associated with the driving. Similarly, you may find yourself feeling upset or emotionally troubled, but may be unaware of the thoughts that led to these feelings. If you are responding in a way that is unhealthy, it is important, first, to become *aware* of your thoughts. Awareness is the first step to seeing if the thoughts are accurate—and if they are not, to change them. Changing inaccurate thoughts leads to changes in feelings and behaviors.

How would you react to the following situation?

Situation: You just ate an extra slice of cake that was not on your meal plan.

What are your *thoughts* about this situation? What are you saying to yourself?

_____

_____

_____

_____

_____

_____

What are your *feelings* about this situation?

_____

_____

_____

_____

_____

_____

How are you *behaving* in this situation? What do you do and/or say?

_____

_____

_____

_____

_____

_____

STYLES OF THINKING

As you become aware of your automatic thoughts, with time, you may also notice that you have particular styles of thinking. There are some styles of thinking that lead to problematic behaviors, including binge eating. The following are examples of styles of thinking that cause problems.

1. *Overgeneralizations*—making up a rule on the basis of one event and applying it to other situations.
   a. Nobody likes me.
   b. I'm never going to be able to control my eating.
   c. I always feel like binge eating.
2. *Catastrophizing*—assuming the worst possible outcome when that isn't supported by objective evidence.
   a. I've eaten more than is on my meal plan—I'm a total failure.
   b. I binged—I've spoiled everything I've done in treatment.
   c. If I gain 1 pound, I will continue to gain more and more weight.
3. *Dichotomizing*—all-or-none, black-and-white thinking.
   a. I've had one bite too much; I might as well binge.
   b. I binged—the entire day is downhill from here.
   c. I'm either in complete control or out of control.
4. *Minimization*—discounting or minimizing the positive when evaluating oneself.
   a. I may have done well today, but it won't matter unless I don't binge all week.
   b. I did well during the presentation at work, but anyone could have done it.
   c. My eyes might be pretty, but it doesn't matter because my legs are still fat.
5. *Rationalization*—finding excuses to engage in an unhealthy behavior.
   a. I'm just tasting the food, so it won't count.
   b. I had a bad day—I deserve to binge.
6. *Mind Reading*—assuming you know what others are thinking without adequate information.
   a. My friend thinks I shouldn't be eating dessert.
   b. These people just looked at me—they're thinking I'm fat.
7. *Self-Fulfilling Prophecy*—making predictions about the outcome of one event and acting in ways to ensure it will come to pass.
   a. I won't be able to control my eating at the party.
   b. I'll always be overweight.

It is important to begin recognizing your particular styles of thinking in response to situations and to begin challenging these thoughts.

HOMEWORK

1. Continue to complete the Eating Behaviors Self-Monitoring Worksheet (Form 1.2).
2. Complete Restructuring Thoughts Worksheet (Form 4.2).
   - Pick a cue that you have identified.
   - Write down corresponding thoughts, feelings, behaviors, and consequences.
   - Note any "styles of thinking" errors.
   - Leave bottom half ("Revised Thoughts," etc.) blank for now; you will complete it after the next session.
3. Read Session 5 Lecture Handout (Form 5.1).
4. Select a goal for the week and a reward:

Goal: _____

Reward: _____

Form 4.2

RESTRUCTURING THOUGHTS WORKSHEET

CUE	RESPONSES		CONSEQUENCES
	THOUGHTS	BEHAVIORS	
	FEELINGS		
	REVISED THOUGHTS	REVISED BEHAVIORS	REVISED CONSEQUENCES
	REVISED FEELINGS		

SESSION 5 LECTURE HANDOUT

Session 5. Restructuring Your Thoughts

In the last session, you learned that it is important to become aware of thoughts and feelings that are linked with your problematic eating. This is the first step to restructuring your thoughts. "Restructuring your thoughts" means changing them. The second step is to evaluate those thoughts. Are they accurate or reasonable? There are two ways that you can determine the accuracy of your thoughts. The first way is to challenge your thoughts by questioning them. The second way is to set up experiments that test the accuracy of your thoughts. After evaluating your problematic thoughts, you can consider revising them. What you would change about your thinking to make it more accurate? The fourth step is to evaluate how your revised thoughts change your feelings, behaviors, and consequences.

STEP 1: IDENTIFY THE CUE AND THE THOUGHTS

Example

Cue: I ate a chocolate chip cookie.

Thoughts: "I'm going to gain weight. I might as well binge-eat. I blew it. The cookie isn't on my meal plan—I've eaten more than I planned to. I'm a failure."

Feelings: Guilt, anxiety, depression.

Behaviors: Binge eating followed by fasting.

Consequences: Feel disgusted and depressed; avoid going to friend's house (social isolation).

STEP 2: EVALUATE YOUR THOUGHTS (EVIDENCE FOR, EVIDENCE AGAINST)

Method 1: Challenging Problematic Thoughts by Questioning Them

Ask yourself if your thoughts are really accurate. The primary questions, which help you to evaluate your thoughts, are:

1. What is the *evidence* for and against my thoughts?
2. What are the *consequences* of my thoughts?

Example

What is the evidence?   For—None.
                         Against—Eating one cookie will not make me gain weight.

What are the   Eating one chocolate chip cookie will *not* ruin my life. It will not lead directly
consequences of   to weight gain. Binge eating will make me feel worse.
the revised thought?

Method 2: Challenging Problematic Thoughts by Testing Them

Another method of challenging thoughts is to test them by setting up experiments to determine their accuracy. For example, suppose that you believe that eating three meals a day will lead to a 10-pound weight gain. The best way to determine whether this is an accurate belief is to actually eat three meals a day for a week and determine whether a weight gain occurred.

How can you test the thought "In order to be liked and successful, I need to lose 10 pounds"? Talk to your friends and coworkers. Would they like you better/think you are more successful if you lost 10 pounds?

Are there any problematic thoughts that you can test? What are these?

How can you go about testing these thoughts?

It is possible that in testing some of these thoughts, some may, in fact, be accurate. For example, most people think of weight as a significant issue. However, the extent to which your weight influences your likeability and success may be exaggerated in your own mind, and the best way for you to be able to control your weight is to learn to eat regular balanced meals. The goal in revising your thoughts is to be both accurate and realistic.

STEP 3: CHANGE YOUR THOUGHTS

Example

What are the revised thoughts?	Even though I have eaten the cookie, it is better not to binge eat since it will set me up for feeling depressed and continuing to binge. It's okay to have a cookie. It does not make me a bad person, and it does not mean I will gain weight. I can modify my meal plan for today.

STEP 4: DETERMINE THE EFFECTS OF YOUR REVISED THOUGHTS

Example

What are the revised feelings?	Less anxious, less depressed.
What are the revised behaviors?	Not binge eating.
What are the revised consequences?	Sense of achievement, sense of being in control; go to friend's house as planned, increased self-esteem.

HOMEWORK

1. Continue to complete the Eating Behaviors Self-Monitoring Worksheet (Form 1.2).
2. Complete the Restructuring Thoughts Worksheet (Form 4.1) as follows:
   - Copy a situation or specific **CUE** that you have listed in Step 1 of your last assignment, as well as the **THOUGHTS, FEELINGS, BEHAVIORS,** and **CONSEQUENCES.**
   - Evaluate and challenge your thoughts or try to test them. Write in these new **THOUGHTS** in the Revised Thoughts section.
   - Now imagine yourself in the same situation (listed under the first column). Given your new way of thinking, how do you think you would respond to this **CUE** or situation now? Write in your new revised **FEELINGS** and **BEHAVIORS** in the appropriate column. What would be the **CONSEQUENCES** of these new responses? Write in the revised **CONSEQUENCES** under the last column.
3. Read Session 6 Lecture Handout (Form 6.1).
4. Select a goal for the week and a reward:

Goal: _____

Reward: _____

SESSION 6 LECTURE HANDOUT

Session 6. Cues and Chains

REVIEW CUE–RESPONSE–CONSEQUENCE SEQUENCE

We have talked about binge-eating behaviors as consisting of five components that create a beginning, middle, and end of a sequence. As shown in the first figure below, the *cue* (beginning) often leads to responses consisting of *thoughts, feelings,* and *behaviors* (middle), which in turn leads to specific *consequences (end).*

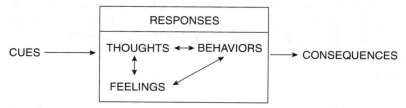

CONSEQUENCES BECOME CUES IN A LONGER BEHAVIORAL CHAIN

But binge-eating behaviors are often more complex than the above sequence suggests. Most of the time, each response or consequence is only one link in a long behavioral chain. For example, a cue such as entering the kitchen after an ample dinner triggers the thought, "I might as well eat more since I already ate too much." This thought becomes the cue that triggers another set of responses, such as feeling agitated. Feeling agitated cues another response, such as opening the refrigerator door, and so on. Writing out a behavioral chain is a helpful strategy for understanding how a particular behavior came about. The figure below illustrates a behavioral chain.

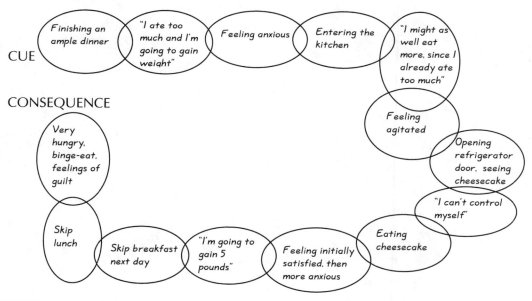

It is very important for you to determine your chain of cues, thoughts, feelings, behaviors, and consequences so that you can break the chain early in the cycle. The earlier the chain is broken, the easier it is to prevent the occurrence of binge eating.

USE CHANGE STRATEGIES TO INTERRUPT THE CHAIN

The strategies for changing behavior that we have already discussed can be used to break a behavioral chain. To review, these strategies include:

Rearranging cues
Avoid or eliminate the cue.
Restrict your stimulus field.
Engage in exposure and response prevention behaviors.

Changing responses to cues:
Build in a pause—delay the response.
Engage in alternative behaviors.
Engage in exposure and response prevention behaviors.

Rearranging consequences:
Structuring response prevention behaviors and rewards.

Changing thoughts
What is the evidence to support or refute my thoughts?
What are the implications of my thoughts?
What are the alternative explanations for my thoughts?
How can I test the accuracy of my thoughts?

Example:

The links in the behavioral chain illustrated on the previous page can be broken by using the various strategies for change: substituting an alternative behavior, avoiding a cue, or restructuring thoughts. Examples of alternative activities include:

Pleasant activities
Calling a friend
Playing the piano
Reading
Necessary activities
Weeding the garden
Vacuuming
Paying bills

Identify and discuss where and how your chains can be broken.

HOMEWORK

1. Continue to complete the Eating Behaviors Self-Monitoring Worksheet (Form 1.2).
2. Complete at least three copies of the Identifying Behavioral Chains Worksheet (Form 6.2), using recent eating binges as the focus.
3. Read Session 7 Lecture Handout (Form 7.1).
4. Select goal for the week and a reward:

Goal: _____

Reward: _____

IDENTIFYING BEHAVIORAL CHAINS WORKSHEET

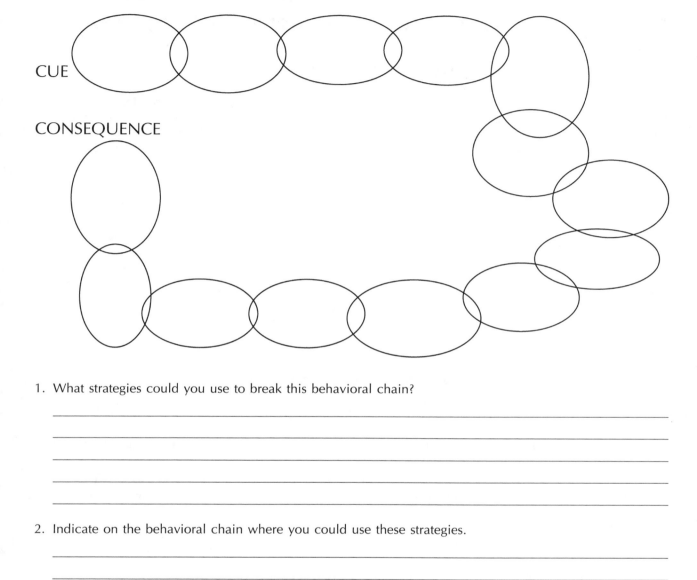

CUE

CONSEQUENCE

1. What strategies could you use to break this behavioral chain?

_____

_____

_____

_____

_____

2. Indicate on the behavioral chain where you could use these strategies.

_____

_____

_____

_____

_____

SESSION 7 LECTURE HANDOUT

Session 7. Impulsivity, Self-Control, and Mood Enhancement

MANAGING YOUR IMPULSES

Binge-eating episodes are often impulsive and unplanned. When you act on impulse, you don't consider the long-term negative consequences. You can learn strategies to reduce impulsive eating and increase self-control. These strategies can help you manage binge eating as well as other problematic behaviors.

Self-control is a learned behavior. People who are impulsive can learn to be more in control of their behaviors.

Consider:

In what situations are you impulsive? _____

_____

_____

What factors affect how impulsive you are (e.g., fatigue, deprivation, anger, intoxication)? _____

_____

STRATEGIES FOR SELF-CONTROL

Greater self-control can be learned by practicing new habits. Some of these new habits include:

- Avoid challenging situations that encourage greater impulsiveness (e.g., drinking alcohol, being alone, attending all-you-can-eat buffets).
- Delay your response by building in a pause. Encourage yourself to wait for some brief period of time before giving in to your impulses. Start with 5 seconds, and over time, increase the delay period. Remember, always choose realistic and attainable goals.
- Self-talk: Talk yourself into staying calm and resisting your immediate impulse.
  1. Verbalize your need to stay calm.
  2. Talk to yourself about preparing for the situation.
  3. Talk to yourself about not giving in to the urge—think about the consequences and remind yourself you have a choice.
  4. Tell yourself to stay calm despite distress, excitement, or arousal.
- Reduce your distress or arousal by:
  1. Deep breathing.
  2. Turning away from the situation and counting backward from 20.
  3. Bringing to mind a calming or distracting image.

- Engage in alternative activities when you begin to feel impulses or urges to eat or at times when you might be most likely to give in to impulsive behavior.
- Exposure-prevention: Place yourself in a situation in which there is some temptation for overeating (or other impulsive behavior) but prevent yourself from doing it, either at all or for some time (delay). This strategy might be best accomplished with a friend—but only a friend who understands that you might still give in to your impulses at some point.

Choose one or more of these approaches to practice this week.

MOOD ENHANCEMENT

Depressed, anxious, and angry moods are often cues for binge-eating episodes. For this reason, managing moods can reduce the likelihood of binge eating.

Understanding the Importance of Pleasant Events

Pleasant events and activities have a strong impact on your mood. If the number of enjoyable activities falls below a critical level, mood becomes depressed. Pleasant activities can be also be "self-nurturing" and serve as a substitute for binge eating. It's important to keep a balance between pleasant activities and neutral or unpleasant events.

Increasing Pleasant Events

You can learn to enhance your mood by maintaining a balance between pleasant and unpleasant activities. You can use pleasant activities as rewards for reaching your goals. However, pleasurable activities are important to schedule regularly for their own sake, aside from their value as rewards. The following four steps can help you increase the pleasant activities you experience as rewards:

1. **Set goals.**
   No goal is too small.
   Don't choose too large a goal because you may set yourself up for failure.
   You can always change your goals to make them more realistic and attainable.
2. **Select rewards for reaching your goals.**
   Rewards should be things that make you feel good and are available (within your control).
   Rewards should be powerful.
   Rewards work best when they are immediately available.
   Identify a menu of 10 rewards of different strengths.
3. **Make a contract.**
   Make a specific written agreement to reward yourself if you accomplish your goal.
4. **Plan ahead.**
   Schedule your pleasant events on a weekly basis, or
   Schedule your pleasant events a day in advance.
   Don't let yourself back out or make excuses.
   Designate the time and place.
   Make a commitment with another person to help you stick to your contract.
   Anticipate problems and try to prevent them from interrupting your pleasant event.

Don't forget to increase pleasant activities by scheduling them for their own sake, not just as rewards. For example:

1. **Schedule time to relax.**
2. **Schedule time to read the newspaper and magazines**.
3. **Schedule time for a walk in the neighborhood.**

Follow-up and Evaluation

During the week, plan to increase your pleasant events. Then keep track of the number of pleasant activities in which you engage and your daily mood ratings. What relationship do you notice between your mood and pleasant activities?

HOMEWORK

1. Continue to complete the Eating Behaviors Self-Monitoring Worksheet (Form 1.2).
2. Complete the Changing Impulsivity Worksheet (Form 7.2).
3. Complete the Pleasant Activities Worksheet (Form 7.3).
4. Read Session 8 Lecture Handout (Form 8.1).
5. Goals: Choose a strategy for managing impulses and practice it for the week.
6. Select a reward for using an impulse control strategy.
7. Plan to increase the number of pleasant activities you experience this week. Then keep track of these activities and rate your mood daily.

Form 7.2

CHANGING IMPULSIVITY WORKSHEET

Pick a situation in which you find you are impulsive:

_____

_____

_____

What strategies can you use to change your impulsivity in this situation?

_____

_____

_____

Form 7.3

PLEASANT ACTIVITIES WORKSHEET

People: List two people with whom you would like to spend more time each week:

1.

2.

Places: List two places where you would like to spend more time:

1.

2.

Things: List two things you do not own that you would like to have and can afford (e.g., book, CD, new shoes):

1.

2.

Activities: List two activities you would like to do more often than you do now:

1.

2.

Form 8.1

SESSION 8 LECTURE HANDOUT

Session 8. Body Image, Part I

WHAT IS BODY IMAGE?

Body image involves how you perceive and experience your body. There are a number of aspects to body image, including:

1. How you see yourself in the mirror
2. How you see your body's parts when looking at them directly
3. The mental picture your have of your body (in the "mind's eye")
4. How your body feels when it is touched
5. How you experience your body spatially (e.g., how much of a bus seat you seem to occupy)
6. How you experience bodily sensations (e.g., hot/cold temperatures, hunger, anger)
7. The thoughts and self-statements you have about your body
8. The feelings you have about your body

In other words, body image refers to different types of bodily experiences and perceptions. All of these different aspects of body image influence each other, and improving your body image can involve any number of them.

WHAT INFLUENCES BODY IMAGE?

Family, Peers, Childhood, and Adult Experiences

Your body image is influenced by the people and events around you, from the past as well as in the present. Events that occurred when you were young can continue to affect how you view your body as an adult. For instance, being teased about appearance by peers or family members as a child may influence how you feel about your body now. Growing up, you were probably also influenced by watching how your role models felt about their bodies. For example, if a sibling, parent, or friend felt negatively about her or his body, you may have learned to feel badly about your own appearance from watching them.

Influences from Culture and Society

Other factors that influence body image are connected with our Western society and culture. Specifically, how people evaluate their bodies often depends on how much they resemble what the society considers the ideal appearance. In our present Western culture, for example, thinness is highly valued as attractive, but this has not always been the case. Researchers found that the average weight of Miss America contestants and winners has decreased over the past decades. In other time periods, larger body sizes were considered more beautiful. The current emphasis on thinness is especially strong for females. For example, by age 18, 80% of American girls have been on a diet.

Unfortunately, the current ideal of thinness is unrealistic for most people. Although messages in the mass media suggest that an individual can achieve any size she or he wants through diet and exercise, the myth does not conform to our biological realities. The pursuit of an unrealistic degree of thinness can result in chronic dieting followed by binge eating, obsessions with body size, and constant dissatisfaction with body shape.

BODY IMAGE AND BINGE-EATING DISORDER

People with binge-eating disorder are often quite dissatisfied with their weight and body shape. Some evidence indicates that people with binge-eating problems are more dissatisfied with their shape compared to others of comparable size who do not have binge-eating problems.

Negative thoughts about weight, shape, and appearance play a role in the onset and maintenance of binge-eating problems. Many people start dieting because of dissatisfaction with their appearance and a belief that they should lose weight. As we have discussed in earlier sessions, severe dieting often precipitates binge-eating episodes. Binge eating leads to negative feelings about appearance, which can trigger further binge eating. Thus, body dissatisfaction can contribute to the vicious cycle of binge-eating patterns.

IMPROVING YOUR BODY IMAGE

How you see and feel about your body will influence how you feel about yourself as a person. An important part of recovery is learning to be more accepting of your own body, regardless of shape and size. Although it might be unrealistic for you to go from hating to loving your body, there are ways to improve your body image:

1. Identify the parts of your body with which you do feel comfortable and focus your thinking on those areas when at all possible.
2. Work toward feeling "neutral" about, or accepting of, those body parts you dislike.
3. Work toward changing negative thoughts about your body. As we have discussed in earlier sessions, changing your thoughts can have powerful effects on your feelings and behaviors. For this reason, targeting your negative thoughts about weight and shape is the most effective way to start to feel more comfortable with your appearance.

We encourage you to explore your thoughts about your body, as well as associated feelings and behaviors. You can use the techniques we have discussed in earlier sessions to change your problematic thoughts.

Currently, how do you feel about your body size and shape?

Do you feel more satisfied with some body parts than others?

How much time do you spend thinking about your physical appearance? For example, how many minutes in an hour do you typically spend thinking about it: 20 minutes? 30 minutes? 45 minutes? 55 minutes?

Do thoughts about your body serve as cues that lead to binge-eating behaviors?

Do you see your body accurately? How do you know you are accurate?

How does your weight and body perception affect your feelings about yourself?

Do changes in your weight and body shape influence your self-evaluation?

How important is your physical appearance to you? Do you value other aspects of yourself?

HOMEWORK

1. Continue to complete the Eating Behaviors Self-Monitoring Worksheet (Form 1.2).
2. Complete the Cultural and Family Influences on Body Image Worksheet (Form 8.2).
3. Complete the Changing Your Thoughts about Your Body Worksheet (Form 8.3).
4. Read Session 9 Lecture Handout (Form 9.1).
5. Select a goal for the week and a reward:

Goal: _____

Reward: _____

CULTURAL AND FAMILY INFLUENCES ON BODY IMAGE WORKSHEET

A. What are some of the messages, rules, and beliefs about your body that you remember hearing from your family and peers? From society and the media?

   1. Example: People will like me better if I am thin.

   2. Example: Body fat is a sign of laziness.

   3.

   4.

   5.

B. Do these messages or beliefs influence how you feel about your body today? Which ones?

   1. Example: Yes, I still believe people will like me better if I am thin.

   2. Example: Yes, if my thighs are fat, it's my fault, it's disgusting, and I'm lazy.

   3.

   4.

   5.

C. How can you change these thoughts to reflect more positive and accurate feelings about yourself?

   1. Example: Although appearance does seem to be important to people, I am a likable person regardless of my size. After all, I don't pick my friends because of the way they look, so why do I assume others will do this to me?

   2. Example: Body fat is normal and is necessary for survival and reproduction. The current ideal of attractiveness is unhealthy and unrealistic. Being overweight is not a sign of laziness.

   3.

   4.

   5.

Form 8.3

CHANGING YOUR THOUGHTS ABOUT YOUR BODY WORKSHEET

Acceptance of your body is a one-day-at-a-time process. You may be aware that on one day you feel fat and unattractive, whereas the next day you feel more comfortable with your appearance, even though your body has not actually changed. These shifts in your body image relate to the things you are saying to yourself. Identifying and changing your negative thoughts about your body are essential in improving your feelings about your appearance.

List frequent negative thoughts about your size and shape.

1. Example: I'm fat.

2.

3.

4.

Now, challenge each of the above thoughts using the techniques we have reviewed in previous sessions (if you have difficulty, try asking another group member for assistance). Try using accurate language to make negative statements more neutral.

1. Example: I'm a size 12. I may feel fat, but I'm within my normal weight range for my height.

2.

3.

4.

Another way to begin feeling more positive about your body is to concentrate on the functions of your body. Ask yourself the following:

What does my body enable me to do?

1. Example: My legs enable me to walk.

2.

3.

4.

What does my body allow me to enjoy?

1. Example: My eyes allow me to see beautiful colors.

2.

3.

4.

SESSION 9 LECTURE HANDOUT

Session 9. Body Image, Part II

CHANGING YOUR THINKING ABOUT YOUR BODY

Most people believe that the only way that they can feel better about their bodies is to change their shape and weight. Weight loss can be an important way of feeling better about yourself. However, it is not the only means. You can start to feel more comfortable with your appearance by changing your thoughts and your self-talk. Consider what you avoid or don't let yourself enjoy because of your shape and weight. Many people find that it helps to question the cultural ideal of beauty, and to expand their own view of attractiveness. Expanding your sense of yourself as a person without overemphasizing shape and weight can also help you feel better about your appearance.

AFFIRMATIONS

Everyone has positive qualities. Sometimes these are difficult to identify when we are not feeling good about ourselves, or we may be uncomfortable with expressing positive thoughts about ourselves because it is something we are not used to doing. Not only is it okay to focus on your positive qualities, it is essential in order to feel better about yourself. Positive self-talk is a skill one can develop through practice.

How you think about and talk to yourself can improve your body image and your self-image.

SUGGESTIONS FOR IMPROVING BODY PERCEPTION

1. Try to expand your appreciation of normal female and male body shapes. Visit an art museum or look through art books to see how "beauty" has been represented in other time periods. Look at pictures of movie stars from the 1940s and 1950s. Imagine how these "beauties" from years ago would be evaluated by current standards of attractiveness. Keep in mind how the notion of the "ideal body" is dependent on specific time periods.

2. Remember how much physical appearance is influenced by your own frame of mind. If you feel better about yourself, it will affect how others view you. Affirmations can be helpful in improving your self-image.

3. Monitor the degree to which your negative feelings about your body relate to your moods. Do you feel "fat" when you are sad about something else? Do you find yourself wanting to be thinner when you are feeling anxious? If so, try expressing some of these feelings directly rather than taking them out on your body. Some ideas: Write in a journal, paint a picture, talk to a close friend, create poetry, make a collage.

4. Wear clothes and accessories that make you feel self-confident. Discard anything that is too small. Pay close attention to what colors make you feel best, what kinds of clothes help you feel most confident, which fabric textures are most comfortable for you.

5. Make a list of the activities you are putting off doing until you have the "perfect " body (e.g., going dancing, buying lingerie). Instead of waiting, try doing some of the activities on your list now. After engaging in these activities, consider if your fantasies about how weight loss would change your life are realistic.

6. Give some serious thought to how much of your energy you would like to devote to your appearance. What are the drawbacks of being obsessed with your body? Can you focus on personal attributes other than your appearance? Do you judge others' weight and shape as harshly as you judge your own? Are there aspects of your life toward which you could redirect your energy, such as social, intellectual, or spiritual growth? Make a list of the different parts of yourself that influence your feelings about yourself as a person. How much does weight/shape affect your self-esteem? Are there other aspects that you value more? We have a choice as individuals in determining how many sociocultural ideals we choose to accept.

7. Don't forget that you are not alone in your pursuit of self-acceptance. Many people struggle with these feelings, and it can be helpful to share your thoughts with others who can support you.

8. Additional ideas: _____

_____

_____

HOMEWORK

1. Continue to complete the Eating Behaviors Self-Monitoring Worksheet (Form 1.2).
2. Complete the Affirmations Worksheet (Form 9.2).
3. Add to list of suggestions for improving body perception (in Form 9.1).
4. Read Session Lecture Handout (Form 10.1).
5. Select goal for the week and a reward:

Goal: _____

Reward: _____

AFFIRMATIONS WORKSHEET

How you think about and talk to yourself can improve your body image and your self-image.

List five positive statements about your body:

1.

2.

3.

4.

5.

Now list five positive statements about yourself that do not relate to your physical appearance (e.g., personality, sense of humor):

1.

2.

3.

4.

5.

If you have difficulty with either part of this exercise, try to think of how your friends and family might describe your positive qualities. You can also ask them for ideas.

Write your affirmations on index cards that you can keep with you to read aloud and silently to yourself throughout the day.

Form 10.1

SESSION 10 LECTURE HANDOUT

Session 10. Self-Esteem

HOW DO YOU DEFINE YOURSELF?

Self-esteem is the way in which a person *evaluates* her- or himself. Self-esteem is only one aspect of self-concept; self-concept is a more general term for how a person defines her- or himself.

Many people with binge-eating problems have low self-esteem; they tend to evaluate themselves in a negative, self-critical manner. Specifically, they exaggerate their weaknesses and minimize their strengths. Self-esteem problems often contribute to binge-eating behaviors; many individuals end up eating to make themselves feel better or as a form of "self-punishment." But people usually end up feeling even worse about themselves after binge eating,

TESTING THE ACCURACY OF NEGATIVE SELF-EVALUATIONS

The techniques described in session 5 for evaluating the accuracy of your thoughts can also be used to test thoughts that contribute to low self-esteem. The first step is to check whether you make "thinking errors" in evaluating yourself

Here are some examples of problematic thoughts related to low self-esteem. Each of these is a type of thinking error:

Thought	**Type of Thinking Error**
"I'm no good"	Overgeneralization
"I'm a failure"	
"I never do anything right"	
"I'm worthless"	
"I can't do it—I'll never do it right"	Catastrophizing
"I did it well, but I should have done it better"	Minimization
"If I don't do well at one thing, it means I'll never be successful"	Black-and-white thinking
"Everybody thinks I'm fat"	Mind reading
"My boss just criticized me— she thinks I'm incompetent"	

You can also challenge and test the accuracy of your thoughts, Ask: What is the evidence? What are alternative explanations? What are the implications? What are ways of testing the accuracy of this thought? In addition, examine the type of language you use in evaluating yourself by completing the Self-Concept Inventory (Form 10.2). Adapted from McKay and Fanning (1987).

THE SELF-CONCEPT INVENTORY

1. Using the Self-Concept Inventory (Form 10.2), write descriptive comments about yourself for each of the categories. Include both positive and negative statements.
2. Now go back through the inventory and separate comments about your strengths from those about weaknesses.
3. Rewrite both the strengths and the weaknesses according to the following guidelines:
   For *strengths:* Use synonyms, adjectives, and adverbs to elaborate.
   For *weaknesses:*
   Use neutral instead of negative words.
   Use accurate language that is specific, not general.
   Find exceptions and corresponding strengths.
4. Write a new self-description, including your revised strengths and weaknesses.
5. Remembering your strengths:
   Daily affirmations: Write your strengths down on 3 × 5 cards and read them several times each day.
   Reminder signs: Place signs in your home or at work to cue you to mentally repeat your affirmations.
   Active integration: Each day, select three strengths from your list and remember situations from the past that exemplify those strengths. Consider as many examples as you can for each strength.

More on Revising Weaknesses

Use Neutral Instead of Negative Words

Go through your list and eliminate all words that have negative connotations—*stupid, lazy, fat, ugly,* and so on. These negative labels have a negative impact on self-esteem, especially if you use them frequently.

Old item	Revised item
"Bad at public speaking"	"It is hard for me to talk in front of large groups. I am more comfortable speaking in smaller groups."

Use Accurate Language

Revise the items in your list so that they are purely descriptive. Focus on the facts.

Old item	Revised item
"Lazy"	"I tend to have more energy in the evenings than in the mornings."

Use Specific Rather Than General Language

Eliminate words such as *everything, always, never,* and *completely.* Rewrite the list so that your description is limited to the particular situation, setting, or relationship.

Old item	Revised item
"Always late"	"Have tendency to take on too many tasks in a day and as a result, sometimes shows up late to meetings at work."

Find Exceptions or Corresponding Strengths

This is an essential step for those items that really make you feel bad about yourself.

Old item	Revised item
"Bossy"	"Like to be in charge"

HOMEWORK

1. Continue to complete the Eating Behaviors Self-Monitoring Worksheet (Form 1.2).
2. Complete the Self-Concept Inventory (Form 10.2).
3. Read Session 11 Lecture Handout (Form 11.1).
4. Note: *Sessions will now be every other week.*

Goal: _____

_____

Reward: _____

Goal: _____

_____

Reward: _____

Form 10.2

SELF-CONCEPT INVENTORY
(ADAPTED FROM McKAY AND FANNING, 1987)

Personality: _____

_____

_____

_____

Elaborate Strengths: _____

Revise Weaknesses: _____

_____

Physical Attributes and Appearance: _____

_____

_____

_____

Elaborate Strengths: _____

Revise Weaknesses: _____

_____

Relationships: _____

_____

_____

_____

Elaborate Strengths: _____

Revise Weaknesses: _____

_____

Form 10.2 *(page 2 of 2)*

Work/school Performance _____

_____

_____

_____

_____

_____

Elaborate Strengths: _____

Revise Weaknesses: _____

_____

SESSION 11 LECTURE HANDOUT

Session 11. Stress Management and Problem Solving

WHAT DO YOU THINK ABOUT STRESS?

The negative effects of stress have often been emphasized, so it is easy to assume that stress is something to be avoided. In reality, stress is natural and essential. It is how we respond to stressful events that determines whether we experience stress in a healthy or unhealthy way. What we tell ourselves about the stressful event play an important part in this.

As you read the following information about stress, evaluate your attitudes about it. How do you perceive stressful events? How do you *choose* to respond to these stressors? How do the consequences of stress affect you?

WHAT IS STRESS?

There are two parts to "stress." The first is the event that puts a demand on you. This is called a "stressor." The second part is the stress response. It involves thoughts, emotions, and physical states that are triggered by the stressor.

Stressors

A stressor is any event that places a demand on you. Stressors can be major, such as moving, losing a significant other, getting married. A stressor can also be minor, such as finding a parking place, completing an assignment, going on a blind date.

Most people recognize major stressors, but they often do not pay much attention to the minor ones. Repeated minor stressors can accumulate and become major.

Do you recognize **YOUR** stressors?

What are some stressors in your life?

1. _____
2. _____
3. _____

Stress Response

The stress response involves thoughts, feelings, behaviors, and physical states that are triggered by a stressor. These responses can be positive or negative. Here are some examples:

Types of stress response	Positive responses	Negative responses
Thoughts	I like a challenge. I can get it done. Relax, I'm doing what I can.	I am incompetent. I must do this per-fectly. I can't handle this.
Feelings	Exhilaration Excitement	Anxious Angry Frustrated Sad
Behaviors	Assertive Productive Task-oriented	Withdrawal Avoiding situations Procrastination
Physical States	Increased pulse rate More strength Increased speech	Knots in stomach Headache Trembling

HOW TO MANAGE STRESS

Managing stress means managing both the **stressor** and your **stress response.** Effective stress management means that the results are positive and you are balanced and healthy.

Managing stress involves at least two tasks. The first task, problem solving, is to manage the stressor. It deals directly with the problem or the stressor that is triggering the stress response. The second task, stress management, focuses on reducing stressors in your life as well as managing your stress response.

Sometimes you will need to deal with the problem first and then manage your stress response to that problem. At other times, you will need to address the stress response first and the problem later. Most often, you will be doing these tasks interchangeably; that is, first dealing with the problem until the stress response gets you out of balance (negative consequences), then managing the stress response until you are back in balance (positive consequences). You will then be in the position to return to solving the problem.

Problem Solving: Managing the Stressor

There are seven steps to solving a problem. It's helpful to start by sorting out your feelings and behaviors from the problem situation itself.

1. Identify your feelings and behaviors.
2. Define the problem.
   What has happened?
   What is upsetting about the situation?
3. Decide what you want as an outcome and establish goals.
   What would I prefer to happen?
4. Generate a number of possible solutions.

5. Evaluate each alternative solution; choose the "best" alternative, considering possible consequences.

　　How useful will this outcome be in solving my problem?

　　How difficult will it be to accomplish it?

　　Do the benefits of this solution outweigh the possible costs?

6. Implement—try out a solution.

7. Review the choice afterward.

　　What were the consequences of my action?

　　Am I satisfied with the results?

　　If not, return to Step 5.

Stress Management: Managing Your Stress Response

Consider the following list of strategies for managing your stress response. Some of these strategies work best when put in place before you encounter a stressor. For example, your stress response will be less extreme and easier to manage if you are in good health, physically and emotionally. Other strategies can help you deal with an already triggered stress response.

Promote General Well-Being by Developing Regular Habits

Eat nutritionally balanced meals and snacks each day.

Exercise regularly (but not excessively).

Sleep adequately and regularly.

Listen to your body and relax when needed.

Provide time for pleasant and rewarding activities in your day (make sure to schedule daily).

Provide time for peaceful solitude, for quiet time alone.

Avoid excessive use of alcohol and caffeinated beverages.

Organize Yourself

Set priorities. (No one can do everything at once. Protect yourself from overload—mental, emotional, physical, and behavioral.)

Structure your time. (Plan your day so that you use your time and energy efficiently. Learn to pace your work and activities.)

Set realistic and practical goals. (Monitor your progress toward these goals.)

Make decisions. (Learn to identify alternatives, evaluate their pros and cons, and choose the alternative that is appropriate for you at that time. Use the problem-solving steps described on the previous page. *Note:* Leaving a decision unresolved is a stressor in itself.)

Establish Relationships

Be emotionally involved with others.

Be exposed to different perspectives or ways of thinking.

Get validation of your feelings and check out your perceptions with people whose feedback you trust and respect.

Through others, have more access to information and resources.

With others, have opportunities to practice skills and receive support and encouragement.

Control Your Environment

Avoid too many changes in your life at any one time.

Shield yourself from stressors when necessary. (Control the amount of stimulation in your environment; avoid too little or too many stressors at one time.)

Create a personal stability zone so that there is someone or something on which you can "fall back."

Remove yourself permanently from the stressor. (Change your environment or the situation—eliminate or avoid the stressful cue.)

Manage Your Thoughts and Feelings (Emotional Responses)

Divert your attention (or detach yourself by becoming mentally involved in another activity or thought).

Examine your expectations or thoughts about your ability to cope with this situation: Are your thoughts reasonable, realistic, and accurate?

Examine the words that you use. The words *should* and *must* are usually associated with unrealistic expectations, especially trying to be *perfect.*

Ask yourself: "What is another way of looking at this situation?"

Ask yourself: "When I put this situation in perspective of my whole day or my whole life, is my trouble worth it?" Keep in mind that this situation reflects only one small aspect of your entire life.

Identify, evaluate, test, and change your problematic thoughts. Develop positive, accurate statements. Get your thoughts to work *for* you rather than *against* you.

Challenge old thinking habits by recognizing the functions that they served in the past and the dysfunctions that they serve in the present.

Learn to let go of a thought, feeling, or behavior when it is appropriate to do so.

Learn to accept what you cannot change.

Manage Your Behaviors and Feelings (Physiological Responses)

"Unwind." (Do a short relaxation exercise, meditate, go for a walk, stretch, take a deep breath, etc.)

"Work off" the stress. (Exercise, garden, play tennis, get involved in another activity, etc.)

"Drain off" the stress by using heat and/or massage. (Take a hot bath or sauna, etc.)

Take time out. (Take some breaks or do something else for a short period of time.)

"Talk out" the stress with another person.

HOMEWORK

1. Continue to complete the Eating Behavior Self-Monitoring Worksheet (Form 1.2).
2. Read Learning to Handle Mistakes (Form 11.2).
3. Read Principles of Acceptance and Self-Acceptance (Form 11.3).
4. Complete the Stress Reduction Experiment Worksheet (Form 11.4).
5. Read Session 12 Lecture Handout (Form 12.1).

Goal: _____

Reward: _____

Goal: _____

Reward: _____

Form 11.2

LEARNING TO HANDLE MISTAKES

1. *Reframing mistakes*
   a. A mistake is anything you do that you later, upon reflection, wish you had done differently
   b. Mistakes can be teachers
   c. Mistakes can be warnings
   d. Loss of spontaneity if you are too worried about mistakes
   e. Allow a quota for mistakes

2. *Developing awareness and responsibility*
   a. Accepting the consequences of your actions
   b. Limits of your own awareness typically due to
      1. Ignorance
      2. Forgetting
      3. Denial
      4. No alternatives
      5. Habits

3. *Understanding the nature of making mistakes*
   a. Everyone will always make mistakes.
   b. No one is perfect.
   c. Mistakes do not change a person's good qualities.
   d. A person is not the same as her or his performance.
   e. People are not bad because they make mistakes.
   f. People who make mistakes do not deserve to be blamed and punished.
   g. The reasons why people make mistakes are:
      1. Lack of skill
      2. Carelessness or poor judgment
      3. Not having enough information
      4. Unsound assumptions
      5. Being tired or ill
      6. Having a different opinion

4. *Forgiving yourself*
   a. You made the only decision you could make, given your needs and awareness at the moment you made it.
   b. You have already paid for your mistake by virtue of its consequences.
   c. Mistakes are unavoidable.

PRINCIPLES OF ACCEPTANCE
AND SELF-ACCEPTANCE

1. Human beings cannot be rated as "good" or "bad" people.

2. Every person has positive and negative qualities.

3. When I focus only on the negative characteristics of someone, I feel worse about him or her.

4. When I focus only on my negative qualities, I feel worse about me.

5. When I think negative thoughts about myself, I get more upset than if I think positive thoughts.

STRESS REDUCTION EXPERIMENT WORKSHEET

Identify a stressor in your life. _____

_____

_____

_____

Choose one technique with which to cope or reduce this stressor. _____

_____

_____

_____

_____

Describe the results of your experiment. _____

_____

_____

_____

_____

_____

SESSION 12 LECTURE HANDOUT

Session 12. Assertiveness

WHAT IS ASSERTIVENESS?

Assertive behavior is the responsible expression of feelings and thoughts without violating your own or another's rights. It is the direct and honest statement of what you do and do not want, communicated through both speech and body language. Assertive behaviors can be used to expand your choices in a variety of situations and to develop communication with others. Assertive communication is respectful to yourself and the other person. Aggressive communication is not respectful to the other person. Passive communication is not respectful to yourself.

HOW SELF-TALK CAN LEAD TO PASSIVE, AGGRESSIVE, OR ASSERTIVE BEHAVIORS

Consider the following examples of passive, aggressive, and assertive thoughts, feelings, and behaviors that take place in a conversation with a group of people at a party. In these examples, particular self-statements lead to passive, aggressive, or assertive behaviors. Evaluate the consequences.

1. Passive

Thoughts (self-statements)	Feelings	Behaviors	Consequences
"My opinion isn't important." "I don't want to sound stupid." "No one is interested in what I have to say."	Anxiety Fear	Avoiding conversation Withdrawing	Avoid making "stupid" remarks. Feel increased anxiety and frustration. Feel increased discomfort and want to leave party—to escape. Urge to binge-eat. Fear of expressing thoughts.

2. Aggressive

"My opinion is the only right one." "These people are stupid."	Frustrated Angry	Yelling Standing too close to others Waving hands	Feel satisfied with expressing opinion. Feel increased anger. Feel alienated from others.

3. Assertive

"My opinion is equally important."	Calm	Talking calmly Maintaining eye contact	Improved self-esteem. Fewer urges to binge-eat.

NONVERBAL COMMUNICATION

Nonverbal communication involves eye contact, body posture, voice tone, position of hands and feet, etc. Give examples of nonverbal communication for each of the following:

  1. Passive behavior: _____
  _____
  _____

  2. Assertive behavior: _____
  _____
  _____

  3. Aggressive behavior: _____
  _____
  _____

SUGGESTED ASSERTIVE SELF-STATEMENTS

"It's okay for me to disagree with other people who feel strongly about their opinion."

"I can tell other people how their negative behavior affects me, and I can give them suggestions for behaving in a different way."

"If I don't tell other people how their negative behavior affects me, I am denying them an opportunity to change their behavior."

"When I stand up for myself, I show that I respect myself, and I gain respect from other people."

"I can choose not to assert myself."

"I'm not responsible for other people's happiness and for solving their problems."

"I can change my mind about something after I've had time to think it over."

"My needs are just as important as someone else's needs."

"If I tell someone 'no' and she or he gets angry, it does not mean that I should have said 'yes' to that person."

"It's okay for me to ask other people for help, even if they might be inconvenienced."

HOMEWORK

1. Continue to complete Eating Behaviors Self-Monitoring Worksheet (Form 1.2).
2. Complete the Thoughts Associated with Assertive and Nonassertive Behavior Worksheet (Form 12.2).
3. Read Session 13 Lecture Handout (Form 13.1).

Goal: _____

Reward: _____

Goal: _____

Reward: _____

THOUGHTS ASSOCIATED WITH ASSERTIVE
AND NONASSERTIVE BEHAVIOR WORKSHEET

Many people learn that standing up for their rights is viewed as not okay. What are some messages or rules about communication that you remember hearing from parents, schools, peers, and the media?

1. _____

2. _____

3. _____

Which of these messages underly how you think today? How do your current thoughts relate to your nonassertive behaviors?

1. _____

2. _____

3. _____

How would you change these thoughts so that your behaviors are more assertive?

1. _____

2. _____

3. _____

What kinds of things can you do to test whether the thoughts associated with your nonassertive behaviors are accurate?

1. _____

2. _____

3. _____

4. _____

SESSION 13 LECTURE HANDOUT

Session 13. Weight Management

WHAT IS A HEALTHY WEIGHT FOR YOU?

As discussed in sessions 8 and 9, our current societal ideal of beauty emphasizes a thin body type with which few people are born. The diet and exercise industries are invested in convincing consumers that any amount of weight loss is possible with the "right" products (e.g., exercise equipment, diet foods), but science indicates that body weight is determined, to a large degree, by genetic factors.

Consider the differences between a healthy weight—for you—and media images of ideal body size. Small amounts of weight loss (e.g., 5–10% of body weight) have been found to have significant benefits on physical health and self-esteem. For these reasons, it is important to determine an ideal weight range that is realistic and healthy.

STRATEGIES FOR MAINTAINING A HEALTHY WEIGHT

Healthy Exercise

Healthy exercise has many benefits:

- It helps you increase and maintain metabolism.
- It helps promote positive mood.
- It is an effective coping strategy for stress, anger, and depression.
- Significant health benefits occur for even limited amounts of regular exercise.

Consider these strategies to maximize the benefits of healthy exercise:

- Start gradually and increase length of time and intensity slowly.
- Make the experience as pleasurable as possible to maximize rewarding properties (e.g., exercise with friends, wear comfortable clothing, exercise outside when the weather is pleasant, determine what type of exercise you enjoy the most, try new exercises).
- Set up a reward schedule for regular exercise. Reward yourself for reaching both small and large goals. For example, reward yourself after each session (e.g., with a bubble bath, massage) and give yourself larger rewards after each week of regular exercise. Some people find graphs useful in maintaining motivation because they visually track the amount and frequency of exercise.
- Try to exercise regularly; in addition, look for small opportunities to increase your activity level (e.g., taking the stairs rather than the elevator).
- Avoid excessive or "compulsive" exercise.
- Evaluate your thoughts and watch out for all-or-nothing thinking (e.g., "If I skip a day, I might as well skip the week").

What You Eat

Consider these strategies to maintain a healthy weight:

- Avoid overly restrictive dieting.
- Reduce and limit foods that are high in fat; try substituting healthier alternatives.
- Experiment with the effect of different food types; for example, some people find that carbohydrates promote satiety and comfortable feelings of fullness.
- Pay attention to differences in "biological" hunger versus urges to eat for emotional or other reasons. In general, try to eat planned meals and snacks. If you find you want to keep eating after or between planned meals and snacks even though you aren't hungry, try an alternative behavior instead.

Don't Put Life "On Hold" Until You Lose Weight

What are your "fantasies" of how your life will be different after you lose weight? _____

_____

_____

_____

How realistic are these fantasies? _____

_____

_____

_____

ACTIVITIES YOU ARE PUTTING OFF UNTIL YOU LOSE WEIGHT WORKSHEET

Write a list of activities, purchases, or risks you are putting off while waiting for weight loss.

1.

2.

3.

4.

5.

6.

7.

Try to incorporate the contents of your list into your life now, rather than waiting for the future.

HOMEWORK

1. Continue to complete Eating Behaviors Self-Monitoring Worksheet (Form 1.2).
2. Complete the Activities You Are Putting Off until You Lose Weight Worksheet (Form 13.2).
3. Complete the High-Risk Foods and Situations Worksheet (Form 13.3).
4. Read Session 14 Lecture Handout (Form 14.1).

Goal: _____

Reward: _____

Goal: _____

Reward: _____

HIGH-RISK FOODS AND SITUATIONS WORKSHEET

LIST OF MY HIGH-RISK FOODS

List your most troublesome foods. That is, list those foods that are high-risk for triggering binge-eating behaviors. Start the list with the least troublesome, and end with the most troublesome, highest-risk food.

1._____ (lowest risk)
2._____
3._____
4._____
5._____
6._____
7._____
8._____
9._____
10._____ (highest risk)

LIST OF MY HIGH-RISK SITUATIONS

List the situations that are high-risk for triggering binge eating (lowest to highest risk). Choose situations that you expect to encounter or be engaged in during the next month.

1._____ (lowest risk)
2._____
3._____
4._____
5._____
6._____
7._____
8._____
9._____
10._____ (highest risk)

SESSION 14 LECTURE HANDOUT

Session 14. Relapse Prevention, Part I: Exposure to High-Risk Foods or Situations

PLANNING TO PREVENT RELAPSE

This session and the next will help you develop a plan to prevent the potential for relapse of your binge-eating behaviors. For your plan, consider the following:

- If you decide to pursue weight loss, incorporate the healthy strategies discussed in the previous session.
- Do as much as possible to handle stress in a healthy way (review the materials presented in session 11 on stress management).
- Practice "exposure" to *high-risk situations* and *high-risk foods.* By *exposure* we mean adding back into your life these high-risk cues, but doing it in a controlled way. The following section explains how.

HOW TO PRACTICE "EXPOSURE" TO HIGH-RISK FOODS AND SITUATIONS

To initially control your binge eating, it was necessary to avoid high-risk cues that triggered binge-eating behavior, such as foods high in sugar or fat. Once your binge eating has decreased, you can begin, gradually, to add back high-risk foods and situations to your daily life. These high-risk cues may still trigger urges to binge—perhaps very strong urges, in some cases. However, by following the four steps below, you can weaken these urges and even make them disappear. In other words, you expose yourself to these high-risk cues successfully—without bingeing. Eventually, the food or the situation stops being a cue for bingeing.

- *Step 1.* You may already have taken this first step, which was part of last session's homework. Make a list of high-risk foods and situations—things that trigger the urge to binge. Arrange this list in order of riskiness for binge eating. Place the lowest-risk foods and situations at the top of the list. The next riskiest is written below that. The highest-risk foods and situations should be at the bottom of the list.
- *Step 2.* Start at the top of your list with your least risky food or situation and plan to "expose" yourself to it. For example, in a meal plan, a piece of pie could be included as a dessert after dinner. As part of planning this exposure, build in structure or sufficient support to guarantee success—so you won't binge eat. For example, be specific about the amount of food you are planning to eat, as well as where and when you want to eat it. If you need the support of another person to give yourself the optimal chance for success, you may choose to eat with a supportive friend. You may want to schedule a pleasurable activity immediately after you eat in order to combat anxiety around the situation and to divert yourself if you have urges to binge-eat. Take note of your feelings after you have accomplished a new task. You may choose to discuss these thoughts and feelings with a friend. You can use Forms 14.4 and 14.5 to plan and record your exposures.

- *Step 3.* Continue to practice exposures with this item on your list until you are comfortable and the riskiness of the item has definitely weakened.

- *Step 4.* Expose yourself to the next higher-risk item on your list. Repeat steps 2 and 3 with that item until you are comfortable and the urges to binge are greatly weakened.

TIPS FOR SUCCESSFUL EXPOSURES

- Certain moods (such as anger) or certain thoughts may make it difficult to expose yourself to a new situation. You may need to delay the exposure until these thoughts or feelings are under control.
- You may choose to continue avoiding a few foods. If so, consider your reasons for doing so.
- If some anxiety occurs after any of these practice sessions, it is important *not* to attempt to reduce the anxiety by using binge eating or unhealthy eating habits. Instead, accept the anxiety and practice an alternative coping behavior (e.g., relaxation, talking with a supportive friend, going for a walk). Remind yourself that the anxiety is only a temporary feeling that will subside with time.

QUESTIONS TO HELP YOUR RELAPSE PLANNING

Why do people relapse?

1. Excessive dieting and not eating regular meals.
2. Stressful events, negative emotions, and self-defeating thoughts.
3. What sort of problems/situations/thoughts might contribute to your relapse?

_____
_____
_____

Consider the definitions of a *lapse* versus a *relapse.* What do you think a relapse is? What is a lapse?

_____
_____
_____

Lapses are expected, temporary slips. They can be used as opportunities to learn and get back on track. A relapse is a more enduring return to frequent problematic behaviors, like binge eating. What can you do if you relapse? Imagine yourself in the following scenario:

You have successfully completed treatment but now have to move to another city. You've been free from binge eating for 5 months and have been eating regular meals and snacks. But you are in a new job and are meeting new people. You start encountering some problems in your life. It is certainly stressful to be in new social situations. You find it increasingly difficult to eat regular meals because of your schedule. You very much want to appear attractive to the people around you and are concerned about your weight. You start skipping meals and begin to binge-eat. Within the period of 1 week you go from healthy eating habits to binge-eating behavior again. You are early in the process of relapse. What are you going to do?

1. What do you need to do in terms of your eating behavior and meal planning?

   _____

   _____

   _____

2. What do you need to do in terms of your thoughts about your weight and shape?

   _____

   _____

   _____

3. What do you need to do in terms of social support?

   _____

   _____

   _____

4. What are the chances that these problems will go away on their own?

   _____

   _____

   _____

5. When should you consider seeking professional help?

   _____

   _____

What overall conclusions can you draw about the process of relapse in terms of its prevention, cause, and management in your life?

_____

_____

_____

_____

_____

_____

HOMEWORK

1. Continue to complete the Eating Behaviors Self-Monitoring Worksheet (Form 1.2).
2. Complete the Relapse Scenario Worksheet (Form 14.2), also using a Restructuring Thoughts Worksheet (Form 4.2).
3. Complete the Lapse Plan and Relapse Plan Worksheet (Form 14.3).
4. Complete the Exposures for High-Risk Foods Worksheet (Form 14.4).
5. Complete the Exposure for High-Risk Situations Worksheet (Form 14.5).
6. Read Session 15 Lecture Handout (Form 15.1).

Goal: _____

Reward: _____

Goal: _____

Reward: _____

RELAPSE SCENARIO WORKSHEET

Write your own scenario of an imaginary relapse.

_____

_____

_____

_____

_____

_____

_____

_____

_____

_____

_____

_____

_____

_____

_____

Using a Restructuring Thoughts Worksheet (Form 4.2), examine the cues, thoughts, feelings, behaviors, and consequences involved in your imaginary relapse.

Form 14.3

LAPSE PLAN AND RELAPSE PLAN WORKSHEET

Lapse Plan: Write a step-by-step plan that you will carry out if a lapse occurs. Focus not only on what you would *do,* but also how you would change your *thoughts.*

1. _____

   _____

2. _____

   _____

3. _____

   _____

4. _____

   _____

5. _____

   _____

6. _____

   _____

Relapse Plan: Write a step-by-step plan that you will carry out if relapse occurs. Again, focus not only on what you would *do,* but also how you would change your *thoughts.*

1. _____

   _____

2. _____

   _____

3. _____

   _____

4. _____

   _____

5. _____

   _____

6. _____

   _____

EXPOSURES FOR HIGH-RISK FOODS WORKSHEET

Exposures for foods #1 and #2 on your list of high-risk foods:

Describe foods:

Describe the problematic response (describe the problematic behaviors this food usually triggers):

1. _____
2. _____
3. _____

Describe any problematic thoughts you may have after eating this food:

1. _____
2. _____
3. _____

Describe your plan—what I will *do:*

1. _____
2. _____
3. _____

How I will deal with my problematic *thoughts:*

1. _____
2. _____
3. _____

Evaluate your plan—consequences:

1. _____
2. _____

Ideas about why your plan did or didn't work:

1. _____
2. _____

List what you would do differently next time:

1. _____
2. _____

Exposures for foods #3 and #4 on your list of high-risk foods:

Describe foods:

Describe problematic response (describe problematic behaviors that this food usually triggers):

1. _____
2. _____
3. _____

Describe any problematic thoughts you may have after eating this food:

1. _____
2. _____
3. _____

Describe your plan—what I will *do:*

1. _____
2. _____
3. _____

How I will deal with my problematic *thoughts:*

1. _____
2. _____
3. _____

Evaluate your plan—consequences:

1. _____
2. _____

Ideas about why your plan did or didn't work:

1. _____
2. _____

List what you would do differently next time:

1. _____
2. _____

EXPOSURES FOR HIGH-RISK SITUATIONS WORKSHEET

Exposures for situations #1 and #2 on your list of high-risk situations:

Describe situations:

Describe problematic response: Describe the problematic behaviors this situation usually triggers:

1. _____
2. _____
3. _____

Describe any problematic thoughts you may have after attempting this situation:

1. _____
2. _____
3. _____

Describe your plan—what I will *do:*

1. _____
2. _____
3. _____

How I will deal with my problematic *thoughts:*

1. _____
2. _____
3. _____

Evaluate your plan—consequences:

1. _____
2. _____

Ideas about why your plan did or didn't work:

1. _____
2. _____

List what you would do differently next time:

1. _____
2. _____

Exposures for situations #3 and #4 on your list of high-risk situations:

Describe situations:

Describe maladaptive response (describe maladaptive behaviors):

1. _____

2. _____

3. _____

Describe any maladaptive thoughts you may have after attempting this situation:

1. _____

2. _____

3. _____

Describe your plan—what I will *do:*

1. _____

2. _____

3. _____

How I will deal with problematic *thoughts:*

1. _____

2. _____

3. _____

Evaluate your plan—consequences:

1. _____

2. _____

Ideas about why your plan did or didn't work:

1. _____

2. _____

List what you would do differently next time:

1. _____

2. _____

SESSION 15 LECTURE HANDOUT

Session 15. Relapse Prevention, Part II

Congratulations on completing the program! As you finish treatment, consider which strategies have been effective for you, and what other changes you would like to make in your life now that your binge eating has improved. It is also important to evaluate the progress that you have made in treatment and to praise yourself for your accomplishments.

RECOGNIZE YOUR PROGRESS, PRAISE YOUR ACCOMPLISHMENTS

What strategies have you learned that have been most helpful?

1. _____
2. _____
3. _____
4. _____
5. _____

How can you continue to use these strategies when treatment has ended?

1. _____
2. _____
3. _____
4. _____
5. _____

Use Form 15.2 to recognize the positive changes you've made over the time of this program.

KEEP PRACTICING THE SKILLS YOU HAVE LEARNED

Now that you are finishing treatment, it is important that you continue to practice what you've learned, applying these skills to new challenges when they occur.

As you continue to recover, focus on building the capacity to confront unexpected stressors with increasing confidence and self-esteem.

Practice the skills that you have learned, such as stress management and problem solving, so that you can employ them at times of crisis.

Use the following strategies in any potentially problematic situations:

- Recognize problematic thinking.
- Challenge and test problematic thinking.
- Evaluate expectations.
- Develop greater acceptance of body size and shape.
- Evaluate the situation and related thoughts at times of stress and manage the situation and your response to it effectively.
- Communicate assertively.
- Rearrange and avoid cues and reward yourself.
- Improve self-esteem.

PLANNING A HEALTHY LIFESTYLE

Many people find that once they have tackled their eating problems, they are ready to face other challenges in their life. In addition, time that was spent binge-eating can now be used in other ways. Continue to develop a support network of family and friends. Develop a healthy positive lifestyle with experiences that are unrelated to food or eating. Consider what a healthy lifestyle is for you, and how you would like to structure your time. Use Form 15.3.

Form 15.2

RECOGNIZE YOUR PROGRESS

Think about the changes you have made in treatment. Compare how you are thinking, feeling, and behaving now to when you started. Make sure to acknowledge your progress.

Positive changes in my thoughts, feelings, and behaviors since I started treatment:

1. _____
2. _____
3. _____
4. _____
5. _____
6. _____
7. _____
8. _____
9. _____
10. _____

Positive changes in my thoughts, feelings, and behaviors that people have noticed in me (ask one or two people close to you who know about your involvement in treatment):

1. _____
2. _____
3. _____
4. _____
5. _____
6. _____
7. _____
8. _____
9. _____
10. _____

Form 15.3

HEALTHY LIFESTYLE PLAN

Hours per week	Describe activities
_____	Work/school
_____	Exercise/physical activity
_____	Time alone, meditation, relaxation
_____	Hobbies and educational pursuits
_____	Social activities
_____	Sleep

References

Abbott, D. W., de Zwaan, M., Mussell, M., Raymond, N. C., Seim, H. C., Crow, S., et al. (1998). On the relationship between binge eating and dietary restraint. *Journal of Psychosomatic Research, 44,* 367–374.

Ackard, D. M., Neumark-Sztainer, D., Story, M., & Perry, C. (2003). Overeating among adolescents: Prevalence and association with weight-related characteristics and psychological health. *Pediatrics, 111,* 67–74.

Adami, G. F., Gandolfo, P., Bauer, B., & Scopinaro, N. (1995). Binge eating in massively obese patients undergoing bariatric surgery. *International Journal of Eating Disorders, 17,* 45–50.

Adami, G. F., Gandolfo, P., & Scopinaro, N. (1996). Binge eating in obesity. *International Journal of Obesity, 20,* 793–794.

Agras, W. S., & Telch, C. F. (1998). The effect of caloric deprivation and negative affect on binge eating in obese binge-eating disordered women. *Behavior Therapy, 29,* 491–503.

Agras, W. S., Telch, C. F., Arnow, B., Eldredge, K., Detzer, M. J., Henderson, J., et al. (1995). Does interpersonal therapy help patients with binge eating disorder who fail to respond to cognitive-behavioral therapy? *Journal of Consulting and Clinical Psychology, 63,* 356–360.

Agras, W. S., Telch, C. F., Arnow, B., Eldredge, K., & Marnell, M. (1997). One-year follow-up of cognitive-behavioral therapy for obese individuals with binge eating disorder. *Journal of Consulting and Clinical Psychology, 65,* 343–347.

Agras, W. S., Telch, C. F., Arnow, B., Eldredge, K., Wilfley, D. E., Raeburn, S. D., et al. (1994). Weight loss, cognitive-behavioral, and desipramine treatments in binge eating disorder: An additive design. *Behavior Therapy, 25,* 225–238.

Alger, S. A., Schwalberg, M. D., Bigaouette, J. M., Michalek, A. V., & Howard, L. J. (1991). Effect of a tricyclic antidepressant and opiate antagonist on binge-eating behavior in normoweight bulimic and obese, binge-eating subjects. *American Journal of Clinical Nutrition, 53,* 865–871.

Alger, S., Seagle, H., & Ravussin, E. (1995). Food intake and energy expenditure in obese female bingers and non-bingers. *International Journal of Obesity and Related Metabolic Disorders, 19,* 11–16.

Allison, K. C., Crow, S. J., Reeves, R. R., West, D. S., Foreyt, J. P., DiLillo, V. G., et al. (2007). Binge eating and night eating in type 2 diabetes mellitus. *Obesity, 15*(5), 1287–1293.

Allison, K. C., Wadden, T. A., Sarwer, D. B., Fabricatore, A. N., Crerand, C. E., Gibbons, L. M., et al.

(2006). Night eating syndrome and binge eating disorder among persons seeking bariatric surgery: Prevalence and related features. *Surgery Obesity and Related Disorders, 2,* 153–158.

American Psychiatric Association (1994). *Diagnostic and statistical manual of mental disorders* (4th ed.). Washington, DC: Author.

American Psychiatric Association. (2000). *Diagnostic and statistical manual of mental disorders* (4th ed., text rev.). Washington, DC: Author.

Anderson, D. A., Williamson, D. A., Johnson, W. G., & Grieve, C. O. (2001). Validity of test meals for determining binge eating. *Eating Behavior, 2,* 105–112.

Antony, M. M., Johnson, W. G., Carr-Nangle, R. E., & Abel, J. L. (1994). Psychopathology correlates of binge eating and binge eating disorder. *Comprehensive Psychiatry, 35,* 386–392.

Appolinario, J. C., Bacaltchuk, J., Sichieri, R., Claudino, A. M., Godoy-Matos, A., Morgan, C., et al. (2003). A randomized, double-blind, placebo-controlled study of sibutramine in the treatment of binge-eating disorder. *Archives of General Psychiatry, 60*(11), 1109–1116.

Arnold, L. M., McElroy, S. L., Hudson, J. I., Welge, J. A., Bennett, A. J., & Keck, P. E. (2002). A placebo-controlled, randomized trial of fluoxetine in the treatment of binge-eating disorder. *Journal of Clinical Psychiatry, 63*(11), 1028–1033.

Balsinger, B. M., Murr, M. M., Poggio, J. L., & Sarr, M. G. (2000). Surgery for weight control in patients with morbid obesity. *Medical Clinics of North America, 84,* 477–489.

Barry, D. T., Grilo, C. M., & Masheb, R. M. (2002). Gender differences in patients with binge eating disorder. *International Journal of Eating Disorders, 31,* 63–70.

Barry, D. T., Grilo, C. M., & Masheb, R. M. (2003). Comparison of patients with bulimia nervosa, obese patients with binge eating disorder, and nonobese patients with binge eating disorder. *Journal of Nervous and Mental Disease, 191,* 589–594.

Basdevant, A., Pouillon, M., Lahlou, N., Le-Barzic, M., & Guy-Grand, B. (1995). Prevalence of binge eating disorder in different populations of French women. *International Journal of Eating Disorders, 18,* 309–315.

Beglin, S. J., & Fairburn, C. G. (1992). What is meant by the term "binge"? *American Journal of Psychiatry, 149,* 123–124.

Berkson, J. (1946). Limitations of the application of fourfold table analysis to hospital data. *Biometrics Bulletin, 2,* 47–53.

Beumont, P. J. V., Garner, D., & Touyz, S. W. (1994). Comments on the proposed criteria for eating disorders in DSM IV. *European Eating Disorders Review, 2,* 63–75.

Binford, R. B., Mussell, M. P., Peterson, C. B., Crow, S. J., & Mitchell, J. E. (2004). Relation of binge eating age of onset to functional aspects of binge eating in binge eating disorder. *International Journal of Eating Disorders, 35,* 286–292.

Black, A. E., Prentice, A. M., Goldberg, G. R., Jebb, S. A., Bingham, S. A., Livingstone, M. B., et al. (1993). Measurements of total energy expenditure provide insights into the validity of dietary measurements of energy intake. *Journal of the American Dietetic Association, 93,* 572–579.

Boan, H., Kolotkin, R. J., Westman, E. C., McMahon, R., & Grant, J. P. (2004). Binge eating, quality of life and physical activity improve after roux-en-Y gastric bypass for morbid obesity. *Obesity Surgery, 14,* 341–348.

Bocchieri-Ricciardi, L. E., Chen, E. Y., Munoz, D., Fischer, S., Dymek-Valentine, M., Alverdy, J. C., et al. (2006). Pre-surgery binge eating status: Effect on eating behavior and weight outcome after gastric bypass. *Obesity Surgery, 16,* 1198–1204.

Bolger, N. (1990). Coping as a personality process: A prospective study. *Journal of Personal and Social Psychology, 59,* 525–537.

Bolger, N., & Zuckerman, A. (1995). A framework for studying personality in the stress process. *Journal of Personality and Social Psychology, 69,* 890–902.

Branson, R., Potoczna, N., Kral, J. G., Lentes, K. U., Hoehe, M. R., & Horber, F. F. (2003). Binge eating as a major phenotype of melanocortin 4 receptor gene mutations. *New England Journal of Medicine, 348,* 1096–1103.

Bray, G. A. (2003). Risks of obesity. *Endocrinology and Metabolism Clinics of North America, 32,* 787–804.

Brody, M. L., Masheb, R. M., & Grilo, C. M. (2005). Treatment preferences of patients with binge eating disorder. *International Journal of Eating Disorders, 37*(4), 352–356.

Brody, M. L., Walsh, B. T., & Devlin, M. J. (1994). Binge eating disorder: Reliability and validity of a new diagnostic category. *Journal of Consulting and Clinical Psychology, 62,* 381–386.

Brolin, R. L., Obertson, L. B., Kenler, H. A., & Cody, R. P. (1994). Weight loss and dietary intake after vertical banded gastroplasty and Roux-en-Y gastric bypass. *Annals of Surgery, 220,* 782–790.

Brownell, K. D. (2002). The environment and obesity. In C. G. Fairburn & K. D. Brownell (Eds.), *Eating disorders and obesity: A comprehensive handbook* (2nd ed., pp. 433–438). New York: Guilford Press.

Brownell, K. D. (2004). *The LEARN program for weight management* (10th ed.). Dallas, TX: American Health.

Bruce, B., & Agras, W. S. (1992). Binge eating in females: A population-based investigation. *International Journal of Eating Disorders, 12,* 365–373.

Bryant-Waugh, R. J., Cooper, P. J., Taylor, C. L., & Lask, B. D. (1996). The use of the Eating Disorder Examination with children: A pilot study. *International Journal of Eating Disorders, 19,* 391–397.

Bryant-Waugh, R., & Lask, B. (1995). Eating disorders in children. *Journal of Child Psychology and Psychiatry and Allied Disciplines, 36,* 191–202.

Bulik, C. M., Sullivan, P. F., & Kendler, K. S. (2000). An empirical study of the classification of eating disorders. *American Journal of Psychiatry, 157,* 886–895.

Bulik, C. M., Sullivan, P. F., & Kendler, K. S. (2002). Medical and psychiatric morbidity in obese women with and without binge eating. *International Journal of Eating Disorders, 32,* 72–78.

Bulik, C. M., Sullivan, P. F., & Kendler, K. S. (2003). Genetic and environmental contributions to obesity and binge eating. *International Journal of Eating Disorders, 33,* 293–298.

Burgmer, R., Grigutsch, K., Zipfel, S., Wolf, A. M., de Zwaan, M., Husemann, B., et al. (2005). The influence of eating behavior and eating pathology of weight loss after gastric restriction operations. *Obesity Research, 15,* 684–691.

Busetto, L., Segato, G., De Luca, M., De Marchi, F., Foletto, M., Vianello, M., et al. (2005). Weight loss and post operative complications in morbidly obese patients with binge eating disorder traeted by laparoscopic adjustable gastric banding. *Obesity Surgery, 15,* 195–201.

Busetto, L., Segato, G., deMarche, F., Foletto, M., de Luca, M., Caniato, D., et al. (2002). Outcome predictors in morbidly obese recipients of an adjustable gastric band. *Obesity Surgery, 12,* 83–92.

Busetto, L., Valente, P., Pisent, C., Segato, G., de Marshi, F., Favretti, F., et al. (1996). Eating pattern in the first year following adjustable silicone gastric banding (AGSB) for morbid obesity. *International Journal of Obesity, 20,* 539–546.

Cachelin, F. M., Striegel-Moore, R. H., Elder, K. A., Pike, K. M., Wilfley, D. E., & Fairburn, C. G. (1999). Natural course of a community sample of women with binge eating disorder. *International Journal of Eating Disorders, 25,* 45–54.

Carter, J. C., & Fairburn, C. G. (1998). Cognitive-behavioral vs. self-help for binge eating disorder: A controlled effectiveness study. *Journal of Consulting and Clinical Psychology, 66,* 616–623.

Cassin, S. E., & von Ranson, K. M. (2005) Personality and eating disorders: A decade in review. *Clinical Psychology Review, 25,* 895–916.

Claudino, A., Duchesne, M., Sichieri, R., Bacaltchuk, J., Oliverira, I., Appolinario, J., et al. (2006, June). *A randomized, placebo-controlled, double-blind trial of topiramate plus cognitive behavior therapy in binge eating disorder.* Paper presented at the International Conference on Eating Disorders, Barcelona, Spain.

Cooke, E. A., Guss, J. L., Kissileff, H. R., Devlin, M. J., & Walsh, B. T. (1997). Patterns of food selection during binges in women with binge eating disorder. *International Journal of Eating Disorders, 22,* 187–193.

Cooper, Z., & Fairburn, C. (1987). The Eating Disorder Examination: A semi-structured interview for the assessment of the specific psychopathology of eating disorders. *International Journal of Eating Disorders, 6,* 1–8.

Cooper, Z., & Fairburn, C. (2003). Refining the definition of binge eating disorder and nonpurging bulimia nervosa. *International Journal of Eating Disorders, 34,* S89–S95.

Cortufo, P., Barretta, V., & Monteleone, P. (1997). An epidemiological study on eating disorders in two high schools in Napels. *European Psychiatry, 12,* 342–344.

Courcoulas, A., Perry, Y., Buenaventura, P., & Luketich, J. (2003). Comparing the outcomes after laparoscopic versus open gastric bypass. *Obesity Surgery, 13,* 341–346.

Crow, S. J., Agras, W. S., Halmi, K., Mitchell, J. E., & Kraemer, H. C. (2002). Full syndromal vs subthreshold anorexia nervosa, bulimia nervosa and binge eating disorder: A multicenter study. *International Journal of Eating Disorders, 32,* 309–318.

Crow, S. J., Kendall, K., Seaquist, E., Praus, B., & Thuras, P. (2001). Binge eating and other psychopathology in Type II diabetes mellitus. *International Journal of Eating Disorders, 30,* 222–226.

Crow, S. J., Mussell, M. P., Peterson, C. B., Mitchell, J. E., & Knopke, A. (1999). Adequacy of prior treatment in patients with bulimia nervosa. *International Journal of Eating Disorders, 25*(1), 29–44.

Crowell, M. D., Cheskin, L. J., & Musial, F. (1994). Prevalence of gastrointestinal symptoms in obese and normal weight binge eaters. *American Journal of Gastroenterology, 89,* 387–391.

de Zwaan, M. (2001). Binge eating disorder and obesity. *International Journal of Obesity, 25,* S51–S55.

de Zwaan, M., Bach, M., Mitchell, J. E., Ackard, D., Specker, S. M., Pyle, R. L., et al. (1995). Alexithymia, obesity, and binge eating disorder. *International Journal of Eating Disorders, 17,* 135–140.

de Zwaan, M., Lancaster, K. L., Mitchell, J. E., Howell, L. M., Monson, N., Roerig, J. L., et al. (2003a). Health related quality of life in morbidly obese patients: Effect of gastric bypass surgery. *Obesity Surgery, 12,* 773–780.

de Zwaan, M., Mitchell, J. E., Crosby, R. D., Mussell, M. P., Raymond, N. C., Specker, S. M., et al. (2005a). Short-term cognitive behavioral treatment does not improve outcome of a comprehensive very-low-calorie diet program in obese women with binge eating disorder. *Behavior Therapy, 36,* 89–99.

de Zwaan, M., Mitchell, J. E., Howell, L. M., Monson, N., Swan-Kremeier, L., & Crosby, R. D. (2003b). Characteristics of morbidly obese patients before gastric bypass surgery. *Comprehensive Psychiatry, 44,* 428–434.

de Zwaan, M., Mitchell, J. E., Howell, L. M., Monson, N., Swan-Kremeier, L., Roerig, J. L., et al. (2002). Two measures of health-related quality of life in morbid obesity. *Obesity Research, 10,* 1143–1151.

de Zwaan, M., Mitchell, J. E., Mussell, M. P., Raymond, N. C., Seim, H. C., Specker, S. M., et al. (2005b). Short-term cognitive behavioral treatment does not improve long-term outcome of a comprehensive very-low-calorie diet program in obese women with binge eating disorder. *Behavior Therapy, 36,* 89–99.

de Zwaan, M., Mitchell, J. E., Seim, H. C., Specker, S. M., Pyle, R. L., Crosby, R. B., et al. (1994). Eating related and general psychopathology in obese females with binge eating disorder (BED). *International Journal of Eating Disorders, 15,* 43–52.

de Zwaan, M., Mitchell, J. E., Swan-Kremeier, L., McGregor, T., Howell, M. L., Roerig, J. L., et al. (2004). A comparison of different methods of assessing the features of eating disorders in post-gastric bypass patients: A pilot study. *European Eating Disorders Review, 12,* 380–386.

de Zwaan, M., Nutzinger, D. O., & Schönbeck, G. (1992). Binge eating in overweight females. *Comprehensive Psychiatry, 33,* 256–261.

de Zwaan, M., Swan-Kremeier, L., Simonich, H., Lancaster, K., Howell, M., Crosby, R., et al. (2007). A *fine-grained analysis of eating behavior 2-years after gastric bypass surgery for morbid obesity.* Manuscript submitted for publication.

Decaluwe, V., & Braet, C. (2003). Prevalence of binge eating disorder in obese children and adolescents seeking weight loss treatment. *International Journal of Obesity and Related Metabolic Disorders, 27,* 404–409.

Decaluwe, V., & Braet, C. (2005). The cognitive behavioural model for eating disorders: A direct evaluation in children and adolescents with obesity. *Eating Behaviors, 6,* 211–220.

Decaluwe, V., Braet, C., & Fairburn, C. G. (2002). Binge eating in obese children and adolescents. *International Journal of Eating Disorders, 33,* 78–84.

Delgado, C., Morales Gorria, M. J., Maruri Chimeno, I., Rodrigues del Toro, C., Benavente Martin, J. L., & Nunez Bahamonte, S. (2002). [Eating behavior, body attitudes and psychopathology in morbid obesity.] *Actas Espanolas de Psiquiatricos, 30,* 376–381.

Devlin, M. J. (2001). Binge-eating disorder and obesity: A combined treatment approach. *Psychiatric Clinics of North America, 24,* 325–335.

Devlin, M. J., Goldfein, J. A., & Dobrow, I. (2003). What is this thing called BED?: Current status of binge eating disorder nosology. *International Journal of Eating Disorders, 34,* S2–S18.

Devlin, M. J., Goldfein, J. A., Flancbaum, L., Bessler, M., & Eisenstadt, R. (2004). Surgical management of obese patients with eating disorders: A survey of current practices. *Obesity Surgery, 14,* 1252–1257.

Devlin, M. J., Goldfein, J. A., Petkova, E., Jiang, H., Raizman, P. S., Wolk, S., et al. (2005). Cognitive behavioral therapy and fluoxetine as adjuncts to group behavioral therapy for binge eating disorder. *Obesity Research, 13*(6), 1077–1088.

Devlin, M. J., Goldfein, J. A., Petkova, E., Liu, L., & Walsh, B. T. (2007). Cognitive behavioral therapy and fluoxetine for binge eating disorder: Two-year follow-up. *Obesity, 15*(7), 1702–1709.

Devlin, M. J., Walsh, B. T., Spitzer, R. L., & Hasin, D. (1992). Is there another binge eating disorder?: A review of the literature on overeating in the absence of bulimia nervosa. *International Journal of Eating Disorders, 11,* 333–340.

Devlin, M. J., Yanovski, S. Z., & Wilson, G. T. (2000). Obesity: What mental health professionals need to know. *American Journal of Psychiatry, 157,* 854–866.

deVries, M. W. (1992). The experience of psychopathology in natural settings: Introduction and illustration of variables. In M. W. deVries (Ed.), *The experience of psychopathology: Investigating mental disorders in their natural settings* (pp. 3–26), New York: Cambridge University Press.

Didie, E. R., & Fitzgibbon, M. (2005). Binge eating and psychological distress: Is the degree of obesity a factor? *Eating Behaviors, 6,* 35–41.

Dunn, E. C., Neighbors, C., & Larimer, M. E. (2006). Motivational enhancement therapy and self-help treatment for binge eaters. *Psychology of Addictive Behaviors, 20,* 44–52.

Dymek, M. P., le Grange, D., Neven, K., & Alverdy, J. (2001). Quality of life and psychosocial adjustment in patients after roux-en-Y gastric bypass: A brief report. *Obesity Surgery, 11,* 32–39.

Eldredge, K. L., & Agras, W. S. (1996). Weight and shape overconcern and emotional eating in binge eating disorder. *International Journal of Eating Disorders, 19,* 73–82.

Eldredge, K. L., Agras, W. S., Arnow, B., Telch, C. F., Bell, S., Castonguay, L., et al. (1997). The effects of extending cognitive-behavioral therapy for binge eating disorder among initial treatment nonresponders. *International Journal of Eating Disorders, 21,* 347–352.

Elfhag, K., & Rössner, S. (2005). Who succeeds in maintaining weight loss?: A conceptual review of factors associated with weight loss maintenance and weight gain. *Obesity Reviews, 6,* 67–85.

Fairburn, C. G., & Beglin, S. J. (1994). The assessment of eating disorders: Interview versus questionnaire. *International Journal of Eating Disorders, 16,* 363–370.

Fairburn, C. G., & Cooper, Z. (1993). The Eating Disorder Examination (12th edition). In C. G. Fairburn & G. T. Wilson (Eds.), *Binge eating: Nature, assessment, and treatment* (pp. 317–360). New York: Guilford Press.

Fairburn, C. G., Cooper, Z., Doll, H. A., Normal, P., & O'Connor, M. E. (2000) The natural course of bulimia nervosa and binge eating disorder in young women. *Archives of General Psychiatry, 57,* 659–665.

Fairburn, C. G., Doll, H. A., Welch, S. L., Hay, P. J., Davies, B. A., & O'Connor, M. E. (1998). Risk factors for binge eating disorder: A community based case-control study. *Archives of General Psychiatry, 55,* 425–432.

Fairburn, C. G., Marcus, M. D., & Wilson, G. T. (1993). Cognitive-behavioral therapy for binge eating and bulimia nervosa: A comprehensive treatment manual. In C. G. Fairburn & G. T. Wilson (Eds.), *Binge eating: Nature, assessment, and treatment* (pp. 361–404). New York: Guilford Press.

Farooqi, I. S., Keogh, J. M., Yeo, G. S. H., Lank, E. J., Cheetham, T., & O'Rahilly, S. (2003). Clinical spectrum of obesity and mutations in the melanocortin 4 receptor gene. *New England Journal of Medicine, 348,* 1085–1095.

Fassino, S., Leombruni, P., Piero, A., Abbate-Daga, G., & Giacomo Rovera, G. (2003). Mood, eating attitudes, and anger in obese women with and without binge eating disorder. *Journal of Psychosomatic Research, 54,* 559–566.

Favaro, A., Ferrara, S., & Santonastaso, P. (2003). The spectrum of eating disorders in young women: a prevalence study in a general population sample. *Psychosomatic Medicine, 65,* 701–708.

Fichter, M. M., Herpertz, S., Quadflieg, N., & Herpertz-Dahlmann, B. (1998). Structured Interview for Anorexic and Bulimic Disorders for DSM-IV and ICD-10: Updated (third) revision. *International Journal of Eating Disorders, 24,* 227–249.

Fichter, M. M., & Quadflieg, N. (2001). The structured Interview for Anorexic and Bulimic Disorders for DSM-IV and ICD-10 (SIAB-EX): Reliability and validity. *European Psychiatry, 16,* 38–48.

Fichter, M. M., & Quadflieg, N. (2005, September). *Long-term course and outcome of BED and BN. Does it differ?* Paper presented at the meeting of the Eating Disorders Research Society, Toronto, ON, Canada.

Fichter, M. M., Quadflieg, N., & Brandl, B. (1993). Recurrent overeating: An empirical comparison of binge eating disorder, bulimia nervosa, and obesity. *International Journal of Eating Disorders, 14,* 1–16.

Fichter, M. M., Quadflieg, N., & Gnutzmann, A. (1998). Binge eating disorder: Treatment outcome over a 6-year course. *Journal of Psychosomatic Research, 44,* 385–405.

Field, A. E., Austin, S. B., Taylor, C. B., Malspeis, S., Rosner, B., Rockett, H. R., et al. (2003). Relation between dieting and weight change among preadolescents and adolescents. *Pediatrics, 112,* 900–906.

Field, A. E., Coakley, E. H., Must, A., Spadano, J. L., Laird, N., Dietz, W. H., et al. (2001). Impact of overweight on the risk of developing common chronic diseases during a 10-year period. *Archives of Internal Medicine, 161*(13), 1581–1586.

First, M. B., Spitzer, R. L., Gibbon, M., & Williams, J. B.W. (1995). *Structured Clinical Interview for DSM-IV Axis I Disorders: Patient Edition* (SCID-P, Version 2). New York: New York State Psychiatric Institute, Biometrics Research.

Fitzgibbon, M. L., Spring, B., Avellone, M. E., Blackman, L. R., Pingitore, R., & Stolley, M. R. (1998). Correlates of binge eating in Hispanic, black, and white women. *International Journal of Eating Disorders, 24,* 43–52.

Fontaine, K. R., & Allison, D. B. (2004). Obesity and mortality rates. In G. A. Bray & C. Bouchard (Eds.), *Handbook of obesity: Etiology and pathophysiology* (2nd ed., pp. 767–786). New York: Marcel Dekker.

Fowler, S. J., & Bulik, C. M. (1997). Family environment and psychiatric history in women with binge eating disorder and obese controls. *Behaviour Change, 14,* 106–112.

Frasure-Smith, N., Lesperance, F., & Talajic, M. (1993). Depression following myocardial infarction: Impact on 6-month survival. *Journal of the American Medical Association, 267,* 515–519.

French, S. A., Jeffery, R. W., Sherwood, N. E., & Neumark-Sztainer D. (1999). Prevalence and correlates of binge eating in a nonclinical sample of women enrolled in a weight gain prevention program. *International Journal of Obesity, 23,* 576–585.

Friederich, H.-C., Schild, S., Schellberg, D., Quenter, A., Bode, C., Hezog, W., et al. (2005). Cardiac parasympathetic regulation in obese women with binge eating disorder. *International Journal of Obesity, 30,* 534–542.

Geliebter, A., Gluck, M. E., & Hashim, S. A. (2004a, April). *Plasma ghrelin concentrations are lower in binge eating disorder.* Paper presented at the American Society for Nutrition Sciences, Washington, DC.

Geliebter, A., Gluck, M. E., & Hashim, S. A. (2005). Plasma ghrelin concentrations are lower in binge-eating disorder. *Journal of Nutrition, 135,* 1326–1330.

Geliebter, A., Hassid, G., & Hashim, S. A. (2001). Test meal intake in obese binge eaters in relation to mood and gender. *International Journal of Eating Disorders, 29,* 488–494.

Geliebter, A., Yahav, E. K., Gluck, M. E., & Hashim, S. (2004b). Gastric capacity, test meal intake, and appetitive hormones in binge eating disorder. *Physiology and Behavior, 81,* 735–740.

Gladis, M. M., Wadden, T. A., Foster, G. D., Vogt, R. A., & Wingate, B. J. (1998a). A comparison of two approaches to the assessment of binge eating in obesity. *International Journal of Eating Disorders, 23,* 17–26.

Gladis, M. M., Wadden, T. A., Vogt, R., Foster, G., Kuehnel, R. H., & Bartlett, S. J. (1998b). Behavioral treatment of obese binge eaters: Do they need different care? *Journal of Psychosomatic Research, 44,* 375–384.

Glinski, J., Wetzler, S., & Goodman, E. (2001). The psychology of gastric bypass surgery. *Obesity Surgery, 11,* 581–588.

Gluck, M. E. (2006). Stress responses and binge eating disorder. *Appetite, 46,* 26–30.

Gluck, M., Geliebter, A., Hung, J., & Yahav, E. (2004). Cortisol, hunger, and desire to binge eat following a cold stress test in obese women with binge eating disorder. *Psychosomatic Medicine, 66,* 876–881.

Golay, A., Laurent-Jaccard, A., Habicht, F., Gachoud, J. P., Chabloz, M., Kammer, A., et al. (2005). Effect of orlistat in obese patients with binge eating disorder. *Obesity Research, 13*(10), 1701–1708.

Goldfein, J. A., Walsh, B. T., LaChaussee, J. L., Kissileff, H. R., & Devlin, M. J. (1993). Eating behavior in binge eating disorder. *International Journal of Eating Disorders, 14,* 427–431.

Goodrick, G. K., Poston, W. S., Kimball, K. T., Reeves, R. S., & Foreyt, J. P. (1998). Nondieting vs. dieting treatment for overweight binge-eating women. *Journal of Consulting and Clinical Psychology, 66,* 363–368.

Gorin, A. A., le Grange, D., & Stone, A. (2003). Effectiveness of spouse involvement in cognitive behavioral therapy for binge eating disorder. *International Journal of Eating Disorders, 33,* 421–433.

Gormally, J., Black, S., Daston, S., & Rardin, D. (1982). The assessment of binge eating severity among obese persons. *Addictive Behavior, 7*(1), 47–55.

Gosnell, B. A., Mitchell, J. E., Lancaster, K. L., Burgard, M. A., Wonderlich, S. A., & Crosby, R. D. (2001). Food presentation and energy intake in a feeding laboratory study of subjects with binge eating disorder. *International Journal of Eating Disorders, 30,* 441–446.

Green, A. E., Dymek-Valentine, M., Pytluk, S., le Grange, D., & Alverdy, J. (2004). Psychosocial outcome of gastric bypass surgery for patients with and without binge eating. *Obesity Surgery, 14,* 975–985.

Greeno, C. G., Wing, R. R., & Shiffman, S. (2000). Binge antecedents in obese women with and without binge eating disorder. *Journal of Consulting and Clinical Psychology, 68,* 95–102.

Grilo, C. M., & Masheb, R. M. (2000). Onset of dieting versus binge eating in outpatients with binge eating disorder. *International Journal of Obesity, 24,* 404–409.

Grilo, C. M., & Masheb, R. M. (2005). A randomized controlled comparison of guided self-help cognitive behavioral therapy and behavioral weight loss for binge eating disorder. *Behavior Research and Therapy, 43,* 1509–1525.

Grilo, C. M., Masheb, R., Brownell, K., & White, M. (2006). Randomized comparison of cognitive behavioral therapy and behavioral weight loss treatments for obese persons with binge eating disorder. *Obesity, 14*(Suppl.), A35.

Grilo, C. M., Masheb, R. M., & Salant, S. L. (2005a). Cognitive behavioral therapy guided self-help and orlistat for the treatment of binge eating disorder: A randomized, double-blind, placebo-controlled trial. *Biological Psychiatry, 57,* 1193–1201.

Grilo, C. M., Masheb, R. M., & Wilson, G. T. (2001) Subtyping binge eating disorder. *Journal of Consulting and Clinical Psychology, 69,* 1066–1072.

Grilo, C. M., Masheb, R. M., & Wilson, G. T. (2005b). Efficacy of cognitive behavioral therapy and fluoxetine for the treatment of binge eating disorder: A randomized double-blind placebo-controlled comparison. *Biological Psychiatry, 57,* 301–309.

Grissett, N. I., & Fitzgibbon, M. L. (1996). The clinical significance of binge eating in an obese population: Support for BED and questions regarding its criteria. *Addictive Behavior, 21,* 57–66.

Guisado, J. A., & Vaz, F. J. (2003). Personality profiles of the morbidly obese after vertical banded gastroplasty. *Obesity Surgery, 13,* 394–398.

Guss, J. L., Kissileff, H. R., Devlin, M. J., Zimmerli, E., & Walsh, B. T. (2002). Binge size increases with body mass index in women with binge eating disorder. *Obesity Research, 10,* 1021–1029.

Hadigan, C. M., Kissileff, H. R., & Walsh, B. T. (1989). Patterns of food selection during meals in women with bulimia. *American Journal of Clinical Nutrition, 50,* 759–766.

Hasler, G., Pine, D. S., Gamma, A., Milos, G., Ajdacic, V., Eich, D., et al. (2004). The associations between psychopathology and being overweight: A 20-year prospective study. *Psychological Medicine, 34,* 1047–1057.

Hay, P. (1998). The epidemiology of eating disorder behaviors: An Australian community based survey. *International Journal of Eating Disorders, 23,* 371–382.

Hay, P., & Fairburn, C. (1998). The validity of the DSM IV scheme for classifying bulimic eating disorders. *International Journal of Eating Disorders, 23,* 7–15.

Hay, P., Fairburn, C., & Doll, H. (1996). The classification of bulimic eating disorders: A community-based cluster analysis study. *Psychological Medicine, 26,* 801–812.

Hebebrand, J., Geller, F., Dempfle, A., Heinzel-Gutenbrunner, M., Raab, M., Gerber, G., et al. (2004). Binge-eating episodes are not characteristic of carriers of melanocortin-4 receptor gene mutations. *Molecular Psychiatry, 9,* 796–800.

Heinberg, L. J., Thompson, J. K., & Matzon, J. L. (2001). Body image dissatisfaction as a motivator for healthy lifestyle change: Is some distress beneficial? In R. H. Striegel-Moore & L. Smolak (Eds.), *Eating disorders: Innovative directions in research and practice* (pp. 215–232). Washington, DC: American Psychological Association.

Herpertz, S., Albus, C., Lichtblau, K., Kohle, K., Mann, K., & Senf, W. (2000). Relationship of weight and eating disorders in Type 2 diabetes patients: A multicenter study. *International Journal of Eating Disorders, 28,* 68–77.

Herpertz, S., Siffert, W., & Hebebrand, J. (2003). Binge eating as a phenotype of melanocortin 4 receptor gene mutations. *New England Journal of Medicine, 349,* 606–609.

Hilbert, A., Tuschen-Caffier, B., & Vögele, C. (2002). Effects of prolonged and repeated body image exposure in binge-eating disorder. *Journal of Psychosomatic Research, 52,* 137–144.

Hill, A. J. (2004). Does dieting make you fat? *British Journal of Nutrition, 92,* S15–S18.

Ho, K. S., Nichaman, M. Z., Tayor, W. C., Lee, E. S., & Foreyt, J. P. (1985). Binge eating disorder, retention, and dropout in an adult obesity program. *International Journal of Eating Disorders, 18,* 291–294.

Hsu, L. K., Benotti, B. N., Dwyer, J., Roberts, S. B., Saltzman, E., Shikors, S., et al. (1998). Nonsurgical factors that influence the outcome of bariatric surgery: A review. *Psychosomatic Medicine, 60,* 338–346.

Hsu, L. K., Betancourt, S., & Sullivan, S. P. (1996). Eating disturbances before and after gastric bypass surgery: A pilot study. *International Journal of Eating Disorders, 19,* 23–24.

Hsu, L. K., Mulliken, B., McDonagh, B., Krupa Das, S., Rand, W., Fairburn, C., et al. (2002).Binge eating disorder in extreme obesity. *International Journal of Obesity and Related Metabolic Disorders, 26,* 1298–1403.

Hsu, L. K., Sullivan, S. P., & Benotti, P. N. (1997). Eating disturbances and outcome of gastric bypass surgery: A pilot study. *International Journal of Eating Disorders, 21,* 385–390.

Hudson, J. I., Lalonde, J. K., Berry, J. M., Pindyck, L. J., Bulik, C. M., Crow, S. J., et al. (2006). Binge eating disorder as a distinct familial phenotype in obese individuals. *Archives of General Psychiatry, 63,* 313–319.

Hudson, J. I., McElroy, S. L., Raymond, N. C., Crow, S., Keck, P. E., Jr., Carter, W. P., et al. (1998). Fluvoxamine in the treatment of binge-eating disorder: A multicenter placebo-controlled, double-blind trial. *American Journal of Psychiatry, 155*(12), 1756–1762.

Hudson, J. I., Pope, H. G., Wurtman, J., Yurgelun-Todd, D., Mark, S., & Rosenthal, N. E. (1988). Bulimia in obese individuals: Relationship to normal-weight bulimia. *Journal of Nervous and Mental Disorders, 176,* 144–152.

Isnard, P., Michel, G., Frelut, M.-L., Vila, G., Falissard, B., Naja, W., et al. (2003). Binge eating and psychopathology in severely obese adolescents. *International Journal of Eating Disorders, 34,* 235–243.

Jeong, S. K., Nam, H. S., Son, M. H., Son, E. J., & Cho, K. H. (2005). Interactive effects of obesity indexes on cognition. *Dementia and Geriatric Cognitive Disorders, 19,* 91–96.

Johnson, J. G., Spitzer, R. L., & Williams, J. B. (2001). Health problems, impairment and illnesses associated with bulimia nervosa and binge eating disorder among primary care and obstetric gynecology patients. *Psychological Medicine, 31,* 1455–1466.

Joiner, T. (1999, November). *Whirlwind taxometric tutorial and application to binge eating disorder.* Presented at the annual meeting of the Eating Disorders Research Society, San Diego, CA.

Jonas, B. S., Franks, P., & Ingram, D. D. (1997). Are symptoms of anxiety and depressoin risk factors for hypertension? *Archives of Family Medicine, 6,* 43–49.

Kabat-Zinn, J. (1990). *Full catastrophe living: Using the wisdom of your body and mind to face stress, pain, and illness.* New York: Dell.

Kalarchian, M. A., Marcus, M. D., Wilson G. T., Labouvie, E. W., Brolin, R. E., & LaMarca L. B. (2002). Binge eating among gastric bypass patients at long-term follow-up. *Obesity Surgery, 12,* 270–275.

Kalarchian, M. A., Wilson, G. T., Brolin, R. D., & Bradley, L. (1999). Effects of bariatric surgery on binge eating and related psychopathology. *Eating and Weight Disorders, 4,* 1–5.

Keefe, P. H., Wyshogrod, D., Weinberger, E., & Agras, W. S. (1984). Binge eating and outcome of behavioral treatment of obesity: A preliminary report. *Behavior Research and Therapy, 22,* 319–321.

Keel, P. K., Fichter, M., Quadflieg, N., Bulik, C., Baxter, M. G., Thornton, L., et al. (2004). Application of a latent class analysis to empirically define eating disorder phenotypes. *Archives of General Psychiatry, 61,* 192–200.

Kenardy, J., Mensch, M., Bowen, K., Green, B., & Walton, J. (2002). Group therapy for binge eating in Type 2 diabetes: A randomized trial. *Diabetic Medicine, 19,* 234–239.

Kenardy, J., Mensch, M., Bowen, K., & Pearson, S. A. (1994). A comparison of eating behaviors in newly diagnosed NIDDM patients and case-matched control subjects. *Diabetes Care, 17,* 1197–1199.

Kilander, L., Nyman, H., Boberg, M., & Lithell, H. (1997). Cogntive function, vascular risk factors and education: A cross-sectional study on a cohort of 70-year-old men. *Journal of Internal Medicine, 242,* 313–321.

Kinzl, J. F., Traweger, C., Trefalt, E., Mangweth, B., & Biebl, W. (1999). Binge eating disorder in females: A population-based investigation. *International Journal of Eating Disorders, 25,* 287–292.

Kolotkin, R. L., Crosby, R. D., Kosloski, K. D., & Williams, G. R. (2001). Development of a brief research measure to assess quality of life in obesity. *Obesity Research, 9,* 102–111.

Kolotkin, R. L., Head, S., & Brookhart, A. (1997). Construct validity of the impact of weight on Quality of Life Questionnaire. *Obesity Research, 5,* 434–441.

Kolotkin, R. L., Westman, E. C., Ostbye, T., Crosby, R. D., Eisenson, H. J., & Binks, M. (2004). Does binge eating disorder impact weight related quality of life? *Obesity Research, 12,* 999–1005.

Kuehnel, R. H., & Wadden, T. A. (1994). Binge eating disorder, weight cycling, and psychopathology. *International Journal of Eating Disorders, 15,* 321–329.

Laederach-Hofmann, K., Graf, C., Horber, F., Lippuner, K., Lederer, S., Michel, R., et al. (1999). Imipramine and diet counseling with psychological support in the treatment of obese binge eaters: A randomized, placebo-controlled double-blind study. *International Journal of Eating Disorders, 26*(3), 231–244.

Lamerz, A., Kuepper-Nybelen, J., Bruning, N., Wehle, C., Trost-Brinkhues, G., Brenner, H., et al. (2005). Prevalence of obesity, binge eating, and night eating in a cross-sectional field survey of 6-year-old children and their parents in a German urban population. *Journal of Child Psychology and Psychiatry, 46,* 385–393.

Lang, T., Hauser, R., Beddeberg, C., & Klaghofer, R. (2002). Impact of gastric banding on eating behavior and weight. *Obesity Surgery, 12,* 100–107.

Laporte, D. J. (1992). Treatment response in obese binge eaters: Preliminary results using a very low calorie diet (VLCD) and behavior therapy. *Addictive Behaviors, 17,* 247–257.

Larsen, F. (1990). Psychosocial function before and after gastric banding surgery for morbid obesity: A prospective psychiatric study. *Acta Psychiatrica Scandinavica, 82,* 1–57.

Larsen, J. K., van Ramshorst, B., Geenan, R., Brand, N., Stroebe, W., & van Doornen, L. J. (2004). Binge eating and its relationship to outcome after laparoscopic adjustable gastric banding. *Obesity Surgery, 14,* 1111–1117.

Larsen, J. K., van Strien, T., Eisinga, R., & Engels, R. (2006). Gender differences in the association between alexithymia and emotional eating in obese individuals. *Journal of Psychosomatic Research, 60,* 237–243.

Latifi, R., Kellum, J. M., De Maria, E. J., & Sugerman, H. J. (2002). Surgical treatment of obesity. In T. A. Wadden & A. J. Stunkard (Eds.), *Handbook of obesity treatment* (pp. 339–356). New York: Guilford Press.

le Grange, D., Gorin, A., Catley, D., & Stone, A. A. (2001). Does momentary assessment detect binge eating in overweight women that is denied at interview? *European Eating Disorders Review, 9*(5), 309–324.

le Grange, D., Gorin, A., Dymek, M., & Stone, A. (2002). Does ecological momentary assessment improve cognitive behavioural therapy for binge eating disorder: A pilot study. *European Eating Disorders Review, 10*(5), 316–328.

Lewinsohn, P. M., Seeley, J. P., Moerk, K. C., & Striegel-Moore, R. H. (2002). Gender differences in eating disorder symptoms in young adults. *International Journal of Eating Disorders, 32,* 426–440.

Linde, J. A., Jeffery, R. W., Levy, R. L., Sherwood, N. E., Utter, J., Pronk, N. P., et al. (2004). Binge eating disorder, weight control self-efficacy, and depression in overweight men and women. *International Journal of Obesity, 28,* 418–425.

Linehan, M. M. (1993a). *Cognitive behavioral treatment of borderline personality disorder.* New York: Guilford Press.

Linehan, M. M. (1993b). *Skills training manual for treating borderline personality disorder.* New York: Guilford Press.

Lowe, M. R., & Caputo, G. C. (1991). Binge eating in obesity: Toward the specification of predictors. *International Journal of Eating Disorders, 10,* 49–55.

Lubrano-Berthelier, C., Dubern, B., Lacorte, J. M., Picard, F., Shapiro, A., Zhang, S., et al. (2006). Melanocortin 4 receptor mutation in a large cohort of severely obese adults: Prevalence, functional classification, genotype–phenotype relationship and lack of association with binge eating. *Journal of Clinical Endocrinology and Metabolism. 91,* 1811–1818.

Maggio, D. A., & Pi-Sunyer, F. X. (2003). Obesity and Type 2 diabetes. *Endocrinology and Metabolism Clinics of North America, 32,* 805–822.

Malone, M., & Alger-Mayer, S. (2004). Binge status and quality of life after gastric bypass surgery: A one-year study. *Obesity Research, 12,* 473–481.

Mannucci, E., Tesi, F., Ricca, V., Pierazzuoli, E., Barciulli, E., Moretti, S., et al. (2002). Eating behavior in obese patients with and without Type 2 diabetes mellitus. *International Journal of Obesity, 26,* 848–853.

Manson, J. E., Skerrett, P. J., & Willett, W. C. (2004). Obesity as a risk factor for major health outcomes. In G. A. Bray & C. Bouchard (Eds.), *Handbook of obesity: Etiology and pathophysiology* (2nd ed., pp. 813–824). New York: Marcel Dekker.

Manwaring, J. L., Hilbert, A., Wilfley, D. E., Pike, K. M., Fairburn, C. G., Dohm, F. A., et al. (2006). Risk factors and patterns of onset in binge eating disorder. *International Journal of Eating Disorders, 39,* 101–107.

Marchesini, G., Natale, S., Chierici, S., Manini, R., Besteghi, L., Di Domizio, S., et al. (2002). Effects of cognitive-behavioural therapy on health-related quality of life in obese subjects with and without binge eating disorder. *International Journal of Obesity, 26,* 1261–1267.

Marcus, M. D. (1993). Binge eating in obesity. In C. G. Fairburn & G. T. Wilson (Eds.), *Binge eating: Nature, assessment, and treatment* (pp. 77–96) New York: Guilford Press.

Marcus, M. D. (1997). Adapting treatment for patients with binge-eating disorder. In D. M. Garner & P. E. Garfinkel (Eds.), *Handbook of treatment for eating disorders* (2nd ed., pp. 484–493). New York: Guilford Press.

Marcus, M. D., & Kalarchian, M. A. (2003). Binge eating in children and adolescents. *International Journal of Eating Disorders, 34,* S47–S57.

Marcus, M. D., Moulton, M. M., & Greeno, C. G. (1995a). Binge eating onset in obese patients with binge eating disorder. *Addictive Behaviors, 20,* 747–755.

Marcus, M. D., Smith, D., Santelli, R., & Kaye, W. (1992). Characterization of eating disordered behavior in obese binge eaters. *International Journal of Eating Disorders, 12,* 249–255.

Marcus, M. D., Wing, R. R., Ewing, L., Kern, E., Gooding, W., & McDermott, M. (1990a). Psychiatric disorders among obese binge eaters. *International Journal of Eating Disorders, 9,* 69–77.

Marcus, M. D., Wing, R. R., Ewing, L., Kern, E., McDermott, M., & Gooding, W. (1990b). A double-blind, placebo-controlled trial of fluoxetine plus behavior modification in the treatment of obese binge-eaters and non-binge-eaters. *American Journal of Psychiatry, 147,* 876–881.

Marcus, M. D., Wing, R. R., & Fairburn, C. G. (1995b). Cognitive treatment of binge eating v. behavioral weight control in the treatment of binge eating disorder. *Annals of Behavioral Medicine, 17,* S090.

Marcus, M. D., Wing, R. R., & Hopkins, J. (1988). Obese binge eaters: Affect, cognitions, and response to behavioral weight control. *Journal of Consulting and Clinical Psychology, 56,* 433–439.

Marcus, M. D., Wing, R. R., & Lamparski, D. M. (1985). Binge eating and dietary restraint in obese patients. *Addictive Behaviors, 10,* 163–168.

Masheb, R. M., & Grilo, C. M. (2000a). Binge eating disorder: A need for additional diagnostic criteria. *Comprehensive Psychiatry, 41,* 159–162.

Masheb, R. M., & Grilo, C. M. (2000b). On the relation of attempting to lose weight, restraint, and binge eating in outpatients with binge eating disorder. *Obesity Research, 8,* 638–645.

Masheb, R. M., & Grilo, C. M. (2002). On the relationship of flexible and rigid control of eating to body mass index and overeating in patients with binge eating disorder. *International Journal of Eating Disorders, 31,* 82–91.

Masheb, R. M., & Grilo, C. M. (2006). Emotional overeating and its association with eating disorder psychopathology among overweight patients with binge eating disorder. *International Journal of Eating Disorders, 39,* 141–146.

Mason, E. E., & Ito, C. (1969). Gastric bypass. *Annals of Surgery, 170,* 329–339.

Mazzeo, S. E., Saunders, R., & Mitchell, K. S. (2005). Gender and binge eating among bariatric surgery candidates. *Eating Behaviors, 7,* 47–52.

McCann, U. D., & Agras, W. S. (1990). Successful treatment of nonpurging bulimia nervosa with desipramine: A double-blind, placebo-controlled study. *American Journal of Psychiatry, 147*(11), 1509–1513.

McCann, U. D., Rossiter, E. M., King, R. J., & Agras, W. S. (1991). Nonpurging bulimia: A distinct subtype of bulimia nervosa. *International Journal of Eating Disorders, 10,* 679–687.

McElroy, S. L., Arnold, L. M., Shapira, N. A., Keck, P. E., Jr., Rosenthal, N. R., Karim, M. R., et al. (2003a). Topiramate in the treatment of binge eating disorder associated with obesity: A randomized, placebo-controlled trial. *American Journal of Psychiatry, 160*(2), 255–261.

McElroy, S. L., Casuto, L. S., Nelson, E. B., Lake, K. A., Soutullo, C. A., Keck, P. E., Jr., et al. (2000). Placebo-controlled trial of sertraline in the treatment of binge eating disorder. *American Journal of Psychiatry, 157*(6), 1004–1006.

McElroy, S. L., Hudson, J. I., Capece, J. A., Beyers, K., Fisher, A. C., & Rosenthal, N. R. (2007). Topiramate for the treatment of binge eating disorder associated with obesity: A placebo-controlled study. *Biological Psychiatry, 61,* 1039–1048.

McElroy, S. L., Hudson, J. I., Malhotra, S., Welge, J. A., Nelson, E. B., & Keck, P. E., Jr. (2003b). Citalopram in the treatment of binge-eating disorder: A placebo-controlled trial. *Journal of Clinical Psychiatry, 64*(7), 807–813.

McElroy, S. L., Kotwal, R., Hudson, J. I., Nelson, E. B., & Keck, P. E. (2004a). Zonisamide in the treatment of binge-eating disorder: An open-label, prospective trial. *Journal of Clinical Psychiatry, 65*(1), 50–56.

McElroy, S. L., Shapira, N. A., Angold, L. M., Keck, P. E., Rosenthal, N. R., Wu, S. C., et al. (2004b). Topiramate in the long-term treatment of binge-eating disorder associated with obesity. *Journal of Clinical Psychiatry, 65,* 1463–1469.

McGuire, M. T., Wing, R. R., Klem, M. L., Lang, W., & Hill, J. O. (1999). What predicts weight regain in a group of successful weight losers? *Journal of Consulting and Clinical Psychology, 67,* 177–185.

McKay, M., & Fanning, P. (1987). *Self-esteem.* Oakland, CA: New Harbinger.

Milano, W., Petrella, C., Casella, A., Capasso, A., Carrino, S., & Milano, L. (2005). Use of sibutramine, an inhibitor of the reuptake of serotonin and noradrenaline, in the treatment of binge eating disorder: A placebo-controlled study. *Advanced Therapy, 22*(1), 25–31.

Miller, P. M., Watkins, J. A., Sargent, R. G., & Rickert, E. J. (1999). Self-efficacy in overweight individuals with binge eating disorder. *Obesity Research, 7,* 552–555.

Miller, W. C. (1999). Fitness and fatness in relation to health: Implications for a paradigm shift. *Journal of Social Issues, 55,* 207–219.

Mitchell, J. E., & Crow, S. (2006). Medical complications of anorexia nervosa and bulimia nervosa. *Current Opinion in Psychiatry, 19*(4), 438–443.

Mitchell, J. E., Crow, S., Peterson, C. B., Wonderlich, S., & Crosby, R. D. (1998). Feeding laboratory studies in patients with eating disorders: A review. *International Journal of Eating Disorders, 24,* 115–124.

Mitchell, J. E., Lancaster, K. L., Burgard, M. A., Howell, L. M., Krahn, D. D., Crosby, R. D., et al. (2001). Long-term follow-up of patients' status after gastric bypass. *Obesity Surgery, 11,* 464–468.

Mitchell, J. E., Mussell, M. P., Peterson, C. B., Crow, S., Wonderlich, S. A., Crosby, R. D., et al. (1999). Hedonics of binge eating in women with bulimia nervosa and binge eating disorder. *International Journal of Eating Disorders, 26,* 165–170.

Molinari, E., Baruffi, M., Croci, M., Marchi, S., & Petroni, M. L. (2005). Binge eating disorder in obesity: Comparison of different therapeutic strategies. *Eating and Weight Disorders, 10,* 154–161.

Molinari, E., Ragazzoni, P., & Morosin, A. (1997). Psychopathology in obese subjects with and without binge-eating disorder and in bulimic subjects. *Psychological Reports, 80,* 1327–1335.

Monteleone, P., Fabrazzo, M., Tortorella, A., Martiadis, V., Steeitella, C., & Maj, M. (2005a). Circulating ghrelin is decreased in non-obese and obese women with binge eating disorder as well as in obese non-binge eating women, but not in patients with bulimia nervosa. *Psychoneuroendocrinology, 30,* 243–250.

Monteleone, P., Matias, I., Martiadis, V., de Petrocellis, L., Maj, M., & di Marzo, A. V. (2005b). Blood levels of the endocanainoid anandamide are increased in anorexia nervosa and in binge-eating disorder, but not in bulimia nervosa. *Neuropsychopharmacology, 30,* 1216–1221.

Monteleone, P., Tortorella, A., Castaldo, E., & Maj, M. (2006). Association of a functional serotonin transporter gene polymorphism with binge eating disorder. *American Journal of Medical Genetics, 141,* 7–9.

Mussell, M. P., Crosby, R. D., Crow, S. J., Knopke, A. J., Peterson, C. B., Wonderlich, S. A., et al. (2000). Utilization of empirically supported psychotherapy treatments for individuals with eating disorders: A survey of psychologists. *International Journal of Eating Disorders, 27*(2), 230–237.

Mussell, M. P., Mitchell, J. E., de Zwaan, M., Crosby, R. D., Seim, H. C., & Crow, S. J. (1996a). Clinical characteristics associated with binge eating in obese females: A descriptive study. *International Journal of Obesity and Related Metabolic Disorders, 20,* 324–331.

Mussell, M. P., Mitchell, J. E., Weller, C. L., Raymond, N. C., Crow, S. J., & Crosby, R. D. (1995). Onset of binge eating, dieting, obesity, and mood disorders among subjects seeking treatment for binge eating disorder. *International Journal of Eating Disorders, 17,* 395–401.

Mussell, M. P., Peterson, C. B., Weller, C. L., Crosby, R. D., de Zwaan, M., & Mitchell, J. E. (1996b). Differences in body image and depression among obese women with and without binge eating disorder. *Obesity Research, 4,* 431–439.

Myers, T. (2005). Psychological management after bariatric surgery. In J. Mitchell & M. de Zwaan (Eds.), *Bariatric surgery: A guide for mental health professionals* (pp. 125–143). New York: Routledge.

National Heart, Lung and Blood Institute. (1992). Obesity and cardiovascular disease risk factors in black and white girls: The NHLBI Growth and Health Study. *American Journal of Public Health, 82,* 1613–1620.

Nauta, H., Hospers, H., Kok, G., & Jansen, A. (2000). A comparison between a cognitive and a behavioral treatment for obese binge eaters and obese non-binge eaters. *Behavior Therapy, 31,* 441–461.

Neumark-Sztainer, D., Wall, M., Guo, J., Story, M., Haines, J., & Eisenberg, M. (2006). Obesity, disordered eating, and eating disorders in a longitudinal study of adolescents: How do dieters fare 5 years later? *Journal of the American Dietetic Association, 106,* 559–568.

Nicholls, D., Charter, R., & Lask, B. (2000). Children into DSM don't go: A comparison of classification systems for eating disorders in childhood and adolescence. *International Journal of Eating Disorders, 28,* 317–324.

Ogden, C. L., Carroll, M. D., & Flegal, K. M. (2003). Epidemiologic trends in overweight and obesity. *Endicrinology and Metabolism Clinics of North America, 32,* 741–760.

Onyike, C. U., Crum, R. M., Lee, H. B., Lyketsos, C. G., & Eaton, W. W. (2003). Is obesity associated with major depression?: Results from the Third National Health and Nutrition Examination Survey. *American Journal of Epidemiology, 158,* 1139–1147.

Papelbaum, M., Appolinario, J. C., Moreira, R. D. O., Ellinger, V. C. M., Kupfer, R., & Coutinho, W. F. (2005). Prevalence of eating disorders and psychiatric comorbidity in a clinical sample of Type 2 diabetes mellitus patients. *Revista Brasileira de Psiquiatria, 27*(2), 135–138.

Pearlstein, T., Spurell, E., Hohlstein, L. A., Gurney, V., Read, J., Fuchs, C., et al. (2003). A double-blind, placebo-controlled trial of fluvoxamine in binge eating disorder: A high placebo response. *Archives of Women's Mental Health, 6*(2), 147–151.

Pekkarinen, T., Koskela, K., Huikuri, K., & Mustajoki, P. (1994). Long-term results of gastroplasty for morbid obesity: Binge-eating as a predictor of poor outcome. *Obesity Surgery, 4,* 248–255.

Pendleton, V. R., Goodrick, G. K., Poston, W. S., Reeves, R. S., & Foreyt, J. P. (2002). Exercise augments the effects of cognitive-behavioral therapy in the treatment of binge eating. *International Journal of Eating Disorders, 31,* 172–184.

Peterson, C. B., Miller, K. B., Crow, S. J., Thuras, P., & Mitchell, J. E. (2005). Subtypes of binge eating disorder based on psychiatric history. *International Journal of Eating Disorders, 38,* 273–276.

Peterson, C. B., Mitchell, J. E., Crow, S. J., Crosby, R. D., & Wonderlich, S. A. (2006, August). *A ran-*

domized comparison trial of group treatment models for binge eating disorder. Paper presented at the annual meeting of the Eating Disorders Research Society, Port Douglas, Queensland, Australia.

Peterson, C. B., Mitchell, J. E., Engbloom, S., Nugent, S., Mussell, M. P., Crow, S. J., et al. (1998a). Binge eating disorder with and without a history of purging symptoms. *International Journal of Eating Disorders, 24,* 251–257.

Peterson, C. B., Mitchell, J. E., Engbloom, S., Nugent, S., Mussell M. P., Crow, S. J., et al. (2001). Self-help versus therapist-led group cognitive-behavioral treatment of binge eating disorder at follow-up. *International Journal of Eating Disorders, 30*(4), 363–374.

Peterson, C. B., Mitchell, J. E., Engbloom, S., Nugent, S., Mussell, M. P., & Miller, J. P. (1998b). Group cognitive behavioral treatment of binge eating disorder: A comparison of therapist-led vs. self-help formats. *International Journal of Eating Disorders, 24,* 125–136.

Picot, A. K., & Lilenfeld, L. R. R. (2003). The relationship among binge severity, personality psychopathology, and body mass index. *International Journal of Eating Disorders, 34,* 98–107.

Pike, K. M., Devlin, M. J., & Loeb, K. L. (2004). Cognitive-behavioral therapy in the treatment of anorexia nervosa, bulimia nervosa, and binge eating disorder. In J. K. Thompson (Ed.), *Handbook of eating disorders and obesity* (pp. 130–162). Hoboken, NJ: Wiley.

Pike, K. M., Dohm, F. A., Striegel-Moore, R. H., Wilfley, D. E., & Fairburn, C. G. (2001). A comparison of black and white women with binge eating disorder. *American Journal of Psychiatry, 158,* 1455–1460.

Pinaquy, S., Chabrol, H., Simon, C., Louvet, J.-P., & Barbe, P. (2003). Emotional eating, alexithymia, and binge eating disorder in obese women. *Obesity Research, 11,* 195–201.

Polivy, J. (1996). Psychological consequences of food restriction. *Journal of the American Dietetic Association, 96,* 589–592.

Polivy, J., & Herman, C. P. (1985). Dieting and binging: A causal analysis. *American Psychologist, 40,* 193–201.

Polivy, J., & Herman, C. P. (1999). Distress and eating: Why do dieters overeat? *International Journal of Eating Disorders, 26,* 153–164.

Pope, H. G., Lalonde, J. K., Pindyck, L. J., Walsh, T., Bulik C. M., Crow, S. J., et al. (2006). Binge eating disorder: A stable syndrome. *American Journal of Psychiatry, 163,* 2181–2183.

Porzelius, L. K., Houston, C., Smith, M., Arfken C., & Fisher, E. (1995). Comparison of a standard behavioral weight loss treatment and a binge eating weight loss treatment. *Behavior Therapy, 26,* 119–134.

Potoczna, N., Branson, R., Kral, J. G., Piec, G., Steffen, R., Ricklin, T., et al. (2004). Gene variants and binge eating as predictors of comorbidity and outcome of treatment in severe obesity. *Journal of Gastrointestinal Surgery, 8,* 971–981.

Powers, P. S., Perez, A., Boyd, F., & Rosemurgy, A. (1999). Eating pathology before and after bariatric surgery: A prospective study. *International Journal of Eating Disorders, 24,* 295–300.

Puhl, R., & Brownell, K. D. (2001). Obesity, bias, and discrimination. *Obesity Research, 9,* 788–805.

Raymond, N. C., de Zwaan, M., Mitchell, J. E., Ackard, D., & Thuras, P. (2002). Effect of a very low calorie diet on the diagnostic category of individuals with binge eating disorder. *International Journal of Eating Disorders, 31,* 49–56.

Raymond, N. C., Mussell, M., Mitchell, J. E., Crosby, R., & de Zwaan, M. (1995). An age-matched comparison of subjects with binge eating disorder and bulimia nervosa. *International Journal of Eating Disorders, 18,* 135–143.

Raymond, N. C., Neumeyer, B., Warren, C. S., Lee, S. S., & Peterson, C. B. (2003). Energy intake patterns in obese women with binge eating disorder. *Obesity Research, 11,* 869–879.

Reas, D. L., Grilo, C. M., Masheb, R. M., & Wilson, G. T. (2005). Body checking and avoidance in overweight patients with binge eating disorder. *International Journal of Eating Disorders, 37,* 342–346.

Reeves, R. S., McPherson, R. S., Nichaman, M. Z., Harrist, R. B., Foreyt, J. P., & Goodrick, G. K. (2001).

Nutrient intake of obese female binge eaters. *Journal of the American Dietetic Association, 101*, 209–215.

Reichborn-Kjennerud, T., Bulik, C. M., Sullivan, P. F., Tambs, K., & Harris, J. R. (2004). Psychiatric and medical symptoms in binge eating in the absence of compensatory behaviors. *Obesity Research, 12*(9), 1445–1454.

Ricca, V., Mannucci, E., Mezzani, B., Moretti, S., Di Bernardo, M., Bertelli, M., et al. (2001). Fluoxetine and fluvoxamine combined with individual cognitive-behaviour therapy in binge eating: A one-year follow-up study. *Psychotherapy and Psychosomatics, 70*, 298–306.

Rieger, E., Wilfley, D. E., Stein, R. I., Marino, V., & Crow, S. J. (2005). A comparison of quality of life in obese individuals with and without binge eating disorder. *International Journal of Eating Disorders, 37*, 234–240.

Riva, G., Bacchetta, M., Baruffi, M., & Molinari, E. (2002). Virtual-reality-based multidimensional therapy for the treatment of body image disturbances in binge eating disorders: A preliminary controlled study. *IEEE Transactions on Information Technology in Biomedicine, 6*, 224–234.

Riva, G., Bacchetta, M., Cesa, G., Conti, S., & Molinari, E. (2003). Six-month follow-up of in-patient experiential cognitive therapy for binge eating disorders. *CyberPsychology and Behavior, 6*, 251–258.

Rossiter, E. M., Agras, W. S., Telch, C. F., & Bruce, B. (1992). The eating patterns of non-purging bulimic subjects. *International Journal of Eating Disorders, 11*, 111–120.

Rowston, W. M., McCluskey, S. E., Gazet, J. C., Lacey, J. H., Franks, G., & Lunch, D. (1992). Eating behavior: The scopinaro operation as modified by Gazet. *Obesity Surgery, 2*, 355–360.

Sabbioni, M. E., Dickson, M. H., Eychmuller, S., Franke, D., Goetz, S., Hurny, C., et al. (2002). Intermediate results of health related quality of life after vertical banded gastroplasty. *International Journal of Obesity and Related Metabolic Disorders, 26*, 277–280.

Safer, D. L., Lively, T. J., Telch, C. F., & Agras, W. S. (2002). Predictors of relapse following successful dialectical behavior therapy for binge eating disorder. *International Journal of Eating Disorders, 32*, 155–163.

Sanchez-Johnsen, L. A., Dymek, M., Alverdy, J., & le Grange, D. (2003). Binge eating and eating-related cognitions and behavior in ethnic diverse obese women. *Obesity Research, 11*, 1002–1009.

Saunders, R. (2004). "Grazing": A high risk behavior. *Obesity Surgery, 14*, 98–102.

Schiffman, S., Hickcox, M., Paty, J. A., Gnys, M., Richards, T., & Kessel, J. D. (1996). Progression from a smoking lapse to relapse: Prediction from abstinence violation effects, nicotine dependence, and lapse characteristics. *Journal of Consulting and Clinical Psychology, 64*, 993–1002.

Schlundt, D. G., Taylor, D., Hill, J. O., Sbrocco, T., Pope-Cordle, J., Kasser, T., et al. (1991). A behavioral taxonomy of obese female participants in a weight-loss program. *American Journal of Clinical Nutrition, 53*, 1151–1158.

Schoeller, D. A., Ravussin, E., Schutz, Y., Acheson, K. J., Baertschi, P., & Jequier, E. (1986). Energy expenditure by doubly labeled water: Validation in humans and proposed calculation. *American Journal of Physiology, 250*, R823–R830.

Schutz, Y., & Jequier, E. (2004). Resting energy expenditure, thermic effects of food, and total energy expenditure. In G. A. Bray & C. Bouchard (Eds.), *Handbook of obesity: Etiology and pathophysiology* (2nd ed., pp. 615–630). New York: Marcel Dekker.

Schwalberg, M. D., Barlow, D. H., Alger, S. A., & Howard, L. J. (1992). Comparison of bulimics, obese binge eaters, social phobics, and individuals with panic disorder on comorbidity across DSM III-R anxiety disorders. *Journal of Abnormal Psychology, 101*, 675–681.

Sherwood, N. E., Jeffery, R. W., & Wing, R. R. (1999). Binge status as a predictor of weight loss treatment. *International Journal of Obesity and Related Metabolic Disorders, 23*, 485–493.

Siqueira, K. S., Apolinario, J. C., & Sichieri, R. (2004). Overweight, obesity, and binge eating in a non-clinical sample of five Brazilian cities. *Obesity Research, 12*, 1921–1924.

Smith, D. E., Marcus, M. D., Lewis, C. E., Fitzgibbon, M., & Schreiner, P. (1998). Prevalence of binge eating disorder, obesity, and depression in a biracial cohort of young adults. *Annals of Behavioral Medicine, 20,* 227–232.

Smolak, L., & Striegel-Moore, R. H. (2001). Challenging the myth of the golden girl: Ethnicity and eating disorders. In R. H. Striegel-Moore & L. Smolak (Eds.), *Eating disorders: Innovative directions for research and practice* (pp. 111–132). Washington, DC: American Psychological Association.

Smyth, J. M., Soefer, M. H., Hurewitz, A., Kliment, A., & Stone, A. A. (1999). Daily psychosocial factors predict levels of diurnal cycles of asthma symptomatolgy and peak flow. *Journal of Behavioral Medicine, 22,* 179–193.

Specker, S., de Zwaan, M., Raymond, N., & Mitchell, J. (1994). Psychopathology in subgroups of obese women with and without binge eating disorder. *Comprehensive Psychiatry, 35,* 185–190.

Spitzer, R. L., Devlin, M. J., Walsh, B. T., Hasin, D., Wing, R., Marcus, M. D., et al. (1991). Binge eating disorder: To be or not to be in DSM IV. *International Journal of Eating Disorders, 10,* 627–629.

Spitzer, R. L., Devlin, M. J., Walsh, B. T., Hasin, D., Wing, R., Marcus, M., et al. (1992). Binge eating disorder: A multisite field trial of the diagnostic criteria. *International Journal of Eating Disorders, 11,* 191–204.

Spitzer, R. L., Stunkard, A., Yanovski, S., Marcus, M. D., Wadden, T., Wing, R., et al. (1993a). Binge eating disorder should be included in DSM-IV: A reply to Fairburn et al.'s "The classification of recurrent overeating: The binge eating disorder proposal." *International Journal of Eating Disorders, 13,* 161–169.

Spitzer, R. L., Yanovski, S., Wadden, T., Wing, R., Marcus, M. D., Stunkard, A., et al. (1993b). Binge eating disorder: Its further validation in a multisite study. *International Journal of Eating Disorders, 13,* 137–153.

Spurrell, E. B., Wilfley, D. E., Tanofsky, M. B., & Brownell, K. D. (1997). Age of onset for binge eating: Are there different pathways to binge eating? *International Journal of Eating Disorders, 21,* 55–65.

Stader, S. R., & Hokanson, J. E. (1998). Psychosocial antecedents of depressive symptoms: An evaluation using daily experiences methodology. *Journal of Abnormal Psychology, 107,* 17–26.

Steffen, R., Biertho, L., Ricklin, T., Piec, G., & Horber, F. F. (2003). Laparoscopic Swedish adjustable gastric banding: A five-year prospective study. *Obesity Surgery, 13,* 404–411.

Stice, E., & Agras, W. S. (1998). Predicting onset and cessation of bulimic behaviors during adolescence: A longitudinal grouping analysis. *Behavior Therapy, 29,* 257–276.

Stice, E., & Agras, W. S. (1999). Subtyping binge eating disordered women along dieting and negative affect dimensions. *Journal of Consulting and Clinical Psychology, 67,* 460–469.

Stice, E., Agras, W. S., Telch, C. F., Halmi, K. A., Mitchell, J. E., & Wilson, G. T. (2001). Subtyping binge eating disordered women along dieting and negative affect dimensions. *International Journal of Eating Disorders, 30,* 11–27

Stice, E., Cameron, R. P., Killen, J. D., Hayward, C., & Taylor, C. B. (1999). Naturalistic weight-reduction efforts prospectively predict growth in relative weight and onset of obesity among female adolescents. *Journal of Consulting and Clinical Psychology, 67,* 967–974.

Stice, E., Presnell, K., & Shaw, H. (2005). Psychological and behavioral risk factors for obesity onset in adolescent girls: A prospective study. *Journal of Consulting and Clinical Psychology, 73,* 195–202.

Stice, E., Presnell, K., & Spangler, D. (2002). Risk factors for binge eating onset in adolescent girls: A 2-year prospective investigation. *Health Psychology, 21,* 131–138.

Stone, A. A., & Shiffman, S. (1994). Ecological momentary assessment (EMA) in behavioral medicine. *Annals of Behavioral Medicine, 16,* 199–202.

Stone, A. A., Smyth, J. M., Pickering, T., & Schwartz, J. (1996). Daily mood variability: Form of diurnal patterns and determinants of diurnal patterns. *Journal of Applied Social Psychology, 26,* 1286–1305.

Striegel-Moore, R. H., Cachelin, F. M., Dohm, F. A., Pike, K. M., Wilfley, D. E., & Fairburn, C. G. (2001). Comparison of binge eating disorder and bulimia nervosa in a community sample. *International Journal of Eating Disorders, 29,* 157–165.

Striegel-Moore, R. H., Dohm, F. A., Kraemer, H. C., Schreiber, G. B., Crawford, P. B., & Daniels, S. R.

(2005). Health services use in women with a history of bulimia nervosa or binge eating disorder. *International Journal of Eating Disorders, 37*(1), 11–18.

Striegel-Moore, R. H., Dohm, F. A., Kraemer, H. C., Taylor, C. B., Daniels, S., Crawford, P. B., et al. (2003). Eating disorders in white and black women. *American Journal of Psychiatry, 106,* 1326–1331.

Striegel-Moore, R. H., Dohm, F. A., Pike, K. M., Wilfley, D. E., & Fairburn, C. G. (2000a). Recurrent binge eating in black American women. *Archives of Family Medicine, 9,* 83–87.

Striegel-Moore, R. H., Dohm, F. A., Pike, K. M., Wilfley, D. E., & Fairburn, C. G. (2002). Abuse, bullying, and discrimination as risk factors for binge eating disorder. *American Journal of Psychiatry, 159,* 1902–1907.

Striegel-Moore, R. H., Dohm, F. A., Solomon, E. E., Fairburn, C. G., Pike, K. M., & Wilfley, D. E. (2000b). Subthreshold binge eating disorder. *International Journal of Eating Disorder, 27,* 270–278.

Striegel-Moore, R. H., & Franko, D. L. (2003). Epidemiology of binge eating disorder. *International Journal of Eating Disorders, 34,* S19–S29.

Striegel-Moore, R. H., Wilson, G. T., Wilfley, D. E., Elder, K. A., & Brownell, K. D. (1998). Binge eating in an obese community sample. *International Journal of Eating Disorders, 23,* 27–37.

Stunkard, A. J. (1959). Eating patterns and obesity. *Psychiatry Quarterly, 33,* 284–295.

Stunkard, A. J., & Allison, K. C. (2003). Binge eating disorder: Disorder or marker? *International Journal of Eating Disorders, 34,* S107–S116.

Stunkard, A. J., Berkowitz, R., Tanrikut, C., Reiss, E., & Young, L. (1996a). *d*-fenfluramine treatment of binge eating disorder. *American Journal of Psychiatry, 153*(11), 1455–1459.

Stunkard, A. J., Berkowitz, R., Wadden, T., Tanrikut, C., Reiss, E., & Young, L. (1996b). Binge eating disorder and the night eating syndrome. *International Journal of Obesity and Related Metabolic Disorders, 20,* 1–6.

Stunkard, A. J., & Messik, S. (1985). The Three-Factor Eating Questionnaire to measure dietary restraint, disinhibition, and hunger. *Journal of Psychosomatic Research, 29,* 71–83.

Tanco, S., Linden, W., & Earle, T. (1998). Well-being and morbid obesity in women: A controlled therapy evaluation. *International Journal of Eating Disorders, 23,* 325–329.

Tanofsky, M. B., Wilfley, D. E., Spurrell, E. B., Welch, R., & Brownell, K. D. (1997). Comparison of men and women with binge eating disorder. *International Journal of Eating Disorders, 21,* 49–54.

Tanofsky-Kraff, M., Cohen, M. L., Yanovski, S. Z., Cox, C., Theim, K. R., Keil, M., et al. (2006). A prospective study of psychological predictors of body fat gain among children at high risk for adult obesity. *Pediatrics, 117,* 1203–1209.

Tanofsky-Kraff, M., & Yanovski, S. Z. (2004). Eating disorder or disordered eating? Non-normative eating patterns in obese individuals. *Obesity Research, 12,* 1361–1366.

Tasca, G. A., Ritchie, K., Conrad, G., Balfour, L., Gayton, J., Lybanon, V., et al. (2006). Attachment scales predict outcome in a randomized controlled trial of two group therapies for binge eating disorder: An aptitude by treatment interaction. *Psychotherapy Research, 16,* 106–121.

Teixeira, P. J., Going, S. B., Houtkeeper, L. B., Cussler, E. C., Metcalfe, L. L., Blew, R. M., et al. (2004). Pretreatment predictors of attrition and successful weight management in women. *International Journal of Obesity, 28,* 1124–1133.

Teixeira, P. J., Going, S. B., Sardinha, L. B., & Lohman, T. G. (2005). A review of psychosocial pre-treatment predictors of weight control. *Obesity Reviews, 6,* 43–65.

Telch, C. F., & Agras, W. S. (1993). The effects of a very low calorie diet on binge eating. *Behavior Therapy, 24,* 177–193.

Telch, C. F., & Agras, W. S. (1996a). Do emotional states influence binge eating in the obese? *International Journal of Eating Disorders, 20,* 271–279.

Telch, C. F., & Agras, W. S. (1996b). The effects of short-term food deprivation on caloric intake in eating-disordered subjects. *Appetite, 26,* 221–234.

Telch, C. F., Agras, W. S., & Linehan, M. S. (2001). Dialectical behavior therapy for binger eating disorder. *Journal of Consulting and Clinical Psychology, 69,* 1061–1065.

Telch, C. F., Agras, W. S., & Rossiter, E. M. (1988). Binge eating increases with increasing adiposity. *International Journal of Eating Disorders, 7,* 115–119.

Telch, C. F., Agras, W. S., Rossiter, E. M., Wilfley, D., & Kenardy, J. (1990). Group cognitive-behavioral treatment for the nonpurging bulimic: An initial evaluation. *Journal of Consulting and Clinical Psychology, 58,* 629–635.

Telch, C. F., & Stice, E. (1998). Psychiatric comorbidity in women with binge eating disorder: Prevalence rates from a non-treatment-seeking sample. *Journal of Consulting and Clinical Psychology, 66,* 768–76.

Tortorella, A., Monteleone, P., del Giudice, E. M., Cirillo, G., Perrone, L., Castaldo, E., et al. (2005). Melancortin-4 receptor molecular scanning and pro-opiomelanocortin R236G variant screening in binge eating disorder. *Psychiatric Genetics, 15,* 161–163.

Troisi, A., di Lorenzo, G., Lega, I., Tesauro, M., Bertoli, A., Leo, R., et al. (2005). Plasma ghrelin in anorexia, bulimia, and binge-eating disorder: Relations with eating patterns and circulating concentrations of cortisol and thyroid hormones. *Neuroendocrinology, 81,* 259–266.

Tseng, M. C., Lee, M. B., Chen, S. Y., Lee, Y. J., Lin, K. H., Chen, P. R., et al. (2004). Response of Taiwanese obese binge eaters to a hospital-based weight reduction program. *Journal of Psychosomatic Research, 57,* 279–285.

Tylka, T., & Subich, L. M. (1999). Exploring the construct validity of the eating disorder continuum. *Journal of Counseling Psychology, 46,* 268–276.

van Hanswijck de Jonge, P., Van Furth, E. F., Lacey, J. H., & Waller, G. (2003). The prevalence of DSM IV personality pathology among individuals with bulimia nervosa, binge eating disorder and obesity. *Psychological Medicine, 33,* 1311–1317.

Wadden, T. A., Foster, G. D., & Letizia, K. A. (1992). Response of obese binge eaters to treatment by behavior therapy combined with very low calorie diet. *Journal of Consulting and Clinical Psychology, 60,* 808–811.

Wadden, T. A., Foster, G. D., Sarwer, D. B., Anderson, D. A., Gladis, M., Sanderson, R. S., et al. (2004). Dieting and the development of eating disorders in obese women: results of a randomized controlled trial. *American Journal of Clinical Nutrition, 80,* 560–568.

Wadden, T. A., Sarwer, D. B., Womble, L. G., Foster, G. D., McGuckin, B. G., & Schimmel, A. (2001). Psychosocial aspects of obesity and obesity surgery. *Surgical Clinics of North America, 81,* 1001–1024.

Wadden, T. A., Womble, L. G., Stunkard, A. J., & Anderson, D. A. (2002). Psychosocial consequences of obesity and weight loss. In T. A. Wadden & A. J. Stunkard (Eds.), *Handbook of obesity treatment* (pp. 144–169). New York: Guilford Press.

Wade, T. D., Bergin, J. L., Tiggemann, M., Bulik, C. M., & Fairburn, C. G. (2006). Prevalence and long-term course of lifetime eating disorders in an adult Australian twin cohort. *Australian and New Zealand Journal of Psychiatry, 40,* 121–128.

Walsh, B. T., & Boudreau, G. (2003). Laboratory studies of binge eating disorder. *International Journal of Eating Disorders, 34*(Suppl.), 530–538.

Walsh, B. T., Hadigan, C. M., Kissileff, H. R., & LaChaussee, J. L. (1992). Bulimia nervosa: A syndrome of feast and famine. In G. H. Anderson & S. H. Kennedy (Eds.), *The biology of feast and famine: Relevance to eating disorders* (pp. 3–30). San Diego, CA: Academic Press.

Walsh, B. T., Kissileff, H. R., Cassidy, S. M., & Dantzic, S. (1989). Eating behavior of women with bulimia. *Archives of General Psychiatry, 46,* 54–58.

Wegner, K. E., Smyth, J. M., Crosby, R. D., Wittrock, D., Wonderlich, S. A., & Mitchell, J. E. (2002). An evaluation of the relationship between mood and binge eating in the natural environment using ecological momentary assessment. *International Journal of Eating Disorders, 32,* 352–361.

Weissman, M. M., Markowitz, J. C., & Klerman, G. L. (2000). *Comprehensive guide to interpersonal psychotherapy*. New York: Basic Books.

Westenhöfer, J. (2001). Prevalence of eating disorders and weight control practices in Germany in 1990 and 1997. *International Journal of Eating Disorders, 29*, 477–481.

Wilfley, D. E., Agras, W. S., Telch, C. F., Rossiter, E. M., Schnieder, J. A., Golomb Cole, A., et al. (1993). Group cognitive-behavioral therapy and group interpersonal psychotherapy for the nonpurging bulimic individual: A controlled comparison. *Journal of Consulting and Clinical Psychology, 61*, 296–305.

Wilfley, D. E., & Crow, S. (2006, August). *Efficacy of sibutramine for the treatment of binge eating disorder: A randomized multi-center placebo-controlled double blind study*. Paper presented at the annual meeting of the Eating Disorders Research Society, Port Douglas, Queensland, Australia.

Wilfley, D. E., Friedman, M. A., Dounchis, J. Z., Stein, R. I., Welch, R. R., & Ball, S. A. (2000a). Comorbid psychopathology in binge eating disorder: Relation to eating disorder severity at baseline and following treatment. *Journal of Consulting and Clinical Psychology, 68*, 641–649.

Wilfley, D. E., MacKenzie, K. R., Welch, R. R., Ayres, V. E., & Weissman, M. M. (2000b). *Interpersonal psychotherapy for group*. New York: Basic Books.

Wilfley, D. E., Pike, K. M., Dohm, F. A., Striegel-Moore, R. H., & Fairburn, C. G. (2001). Bias in binge eating disorder: How representative are recruited clinical samples? *Journal of Consulting and Clinical Psychology, 69*, 383–388.

Wilfley, D. E., Schwartz, M. B., Spurrell, E. B., & Fairburn, C. G. (2000c). Using the Eating Disorder Examination to identify the specific psychopathology of binge eating disorder. *International Journal of Eating Disorders, 27*, 259–269.

Wilfley, D. E., Welch, R. R., Stein, R. I., Spurrell, E. B., Cohen, L. R., Saelens, B. E., et al. (2002). A randomized comparison of group cognitive-behavioral therapy and group interpersonal psychotherapy for the treatment of overweight individuals with binge eating disorder. *Archives of General Psychiatry, 59*, 713–721.

Wilfley, D. E., Wilson, G. T., & Agras, W. S. (2003). The clinical significance of binge eating disorder. *International Journal of Eating Disorders, 34*, S96–S106.

Williamson, D. A., Gleaves, D. H., & Stewart, T. M. (2005). Categorical versus dimensional models of eating disorders: An examination of the evidence. *International Journal of Eating Disorders, 37*, 1–10.

Williamson, D. A., & Martin, C. K. (1999). Binge eating disorder: A review of the literature after publication of DSM-IV. *Eating and Weight Disorders, 4*, 103–114.

Williamson, D. A., Womble, L. G., Smeets, M. A. M., Netemeyer, R. G., Thaw, J. M., Kutlesic, V., et al. (2002). Latent structure of eating disorder symptoms: A factor analytic and taxometric investigation. *American Journal of Psychiatry, 159*, 412–418.

Wilson, G. T., Nonas, C. A., & Rosenblum, G. D. (1993). Assessment of binge eating in obese patients. *International Journal of Eating Disorders, 13*, 25–33.

Wiser, S., & Telch, C. F. (1999). Dialectical behavior therapy for binge-eating disorder. *Journal of Clinical Psychology, 55*, 755–768.

Wonderlich, S. A., de Zwaan, M., Mitchell, J. E., Peterson, C., & Crow, S. (2003). Psychological and dietary treatments of binge eating disorder: Conceptual implications. *International Journal of Eating Disorders, 34*, S58–S73.

World Health Organization. (1992). *ICD-10 classification of mental and behavioural disorders. Clinical descriptions and diagnostic guidelines*. Geneva: Author.

Yanovski, S. Z. (1993). Binge eating disorder: Current knowledge and future directions. *Obesity Research, 1*, 306–324.

Yanovski, S. Z. (1995). The chicken or the egg: Binge eating disorder and dietary restraint. *Appetite, 24*, 258.

Yanovski, S. Z., Gormally, J. F., Leser, M. S., Gwirtsman, H. E., & Yanovski, J. A. (1994). Binge eating disorder affects outcome of comprehensive very low calorie diet treatment. *Obesity Research, 2,* 205–212.

Yanovski, S. Z., Leet, M., Flood, M., Yanovski, J. A., Gold, P. W., Kissileff, H. R., et al. (1992). Food intake and selection of obese women with and without binge eating disorder. *American Journal of Clinical Nutrition, 56,* 975–980.

Yanovski, S. Z., Nelson, J. E., Dubbert, B. K., & Spitzer, R. L. (1993). Association of binge eating disorder and psychiatric comorbidity in obese subjects. *American Journal of Psychiatry, 150,* 1472–1479.

Yanovski, S. Z., & Sebring, N. G. (1994). Recorded food intake of obese women with binge eating disorder before and after weight loss. *International Journal of Eating Disorders, 15,* 135–150.

Index

Activities You Are Putting Off until You Lose Weight
  Worksheet, 174
Adherence to weight loss treatment, 15
Affective functioning
  alexithymia in BED, 18
  BED comorbid psychopathology and, 20, 21–22
  binge eating to regulate negative emotions, 15, 22,
    36–37, 38
  etiological model of BED, 15
  network of responses, 78
Affirmations Worksheet, 99–100, 154
Age
  BED onset patterns, 13–15
  obese subjects with BED, 9
  presentation for treatment, 17
Alexithymia, obesity in BED and, 18
Alternative to Binge-Eating Worksheet, 85, 86, 114,
    117
Anandamide, 38
Anorexia nervosa
  BED comorbidity, 21
  natural course of BED, 16, 17
  versus BED, 17, 22
Antidepressant therapy, 42–44, 48, 68
Anxiety
  BED comorbidity, 21
  binge eating and, 15
Assertiveness, 104, 168–171
Assessment
  bariatric surgery, 52–53
  calorie intake, 36, 37
  children and adolescents, 11
  client-specific model of BED maintenance, 60–61
  dietary restraint, 13

distress, 6
interview instruments, 4–5. *See also* Self-Concept
    Inventory
patient self-monitoring, 80–81
patient skills for cognitive-behavioral techniques, 77
Atypical binge eating, 4
Automatic thoughts, 62, 131
Avoidant personality disorder, 22

Bariatric surgery
  assessment for, 52–53
  binge-eating behavior before and after, 53–57
  complications, 51
  procedures, 50–52
  psychosocial intervention with, 57
  rationale, 49–50
  weight loss outcomes, 51, 55
BED. *See* Binge-eating disorder
Behavioral therapy
  weight control, 64, 65, 67
  weight loss treatment, 32, 33
  See also Cognitive-behavioral therapy
Binge-eating behavior
  bariatric surgery and, 53–57
  in BED, 35–38, 59–60
  conceptual model for cognitive-behavioral therapy,
    77–80
  dieting and, 124
  hedonics, 18
  intervention to prevent obesity, 15, 26, 33
  leading to obesity, 28–29
  obesity and, 25, 26, 27
  obesity leading to, 30
  onset patterns of BED, 13–15

Binge-eating behavior *(cont.)*
 to regulate emotion, 15, 22, 36–37, 38
 research needs, 70–71
 severity of BED, 65
 weight cycling, 29
 weight loss treatment and, 15, 33
 See also Patterns of overeating
Binge-eating disorder (BED)
 binge-eating behavior in, 35–38, 59–60
 body image and, 148
 clinical conceptualization, 3, 7–9, 12, 26, 70–71
 comorbidity. *See* Comorbidity in BED
 diagnostic criteria, 3–7, 12, 35
 epidemiology, 9–10, 12
 etiology, 13, 15
 medical complications, 39–41, 48
 natural course, 16–17, 22
 normal weight individuals with, 25
 obesity and. *See* Obesity and BED
 onset, 13–15
 patient education, 112–113
 psychobiology, 38–39, 71
 risk factors, 7
BN. *See* Bulimia nervosa
Body image
 BED and, 17, 148
 Cognitive-behavioral therapy, 76, 98–100, 147–154
 determinants, 147–148
 etiological models of BED, 15
 racial differences, 10
 subjective obesity, 58
 therapeutic intervention, 67
Borderline personality disorder, BED comorbidity, 22
Bulimia nervosa (BN), 3–4
 BED comorbidity and, 21–22
 calorie consumption in binge eating, 13
 clinical course, 16
 differential diagnosis, 6
 natural course of BED, 16, 17
 nonpurging, 6–7
 versus BED, 17–18, 22, 70–71

Calorie consumption
 in binge eating, 13, 29, 36, 37
 in obesity, 9, 24
 positive energy balance, 29
Cannabinoids, 38
Changing Impulsivity Worksheet, 145
Changing Thoughts About Your Body Worksheet, 151
Children and adolescents, BED in
 diagnosis, 11
 epidemiology, 10

experiential risk factors, 7
 obesity and, 10, 11
 onset, 13–15
 presentation, 10–11
Citalopram, 44
Cognitive-behavioral therapy
 assertiveness training, 104, 168–171
 augmentation strategies, 67
 behavioral component, 62
 body image intervention, 76, 98–100, 147–154
 client-specific model of BED maintenance, 60–61
 clinician resources, 81
 cognitive component, 62–63, 130–133, 135–137
 conceptual approach to BED, 59, 77–80
 educational component, 61, 85–86, 111–117
 effectiveness, 65, 67, 75
 experiential learning in, 63
 guidelines, 81
 healthy eating recommendations, 125, 173
 healthy lifestyle counseling, 61
 homework assignments, 61, 76, 77, 86
 indications, 76
 model program for BED, 75
 patient resistance, 77
 patient role in treatment planning, 60
 patient self-monitoring in, 61, 80–81
 patient skills for, 77
 with pharmacotherapy, 46, 68, 69
 phases, 76
 relapse prevention, 63, 76, 106–108, 176–188
 session 1
  content and goals, 85–86
  lecture handout, 111–117
 session 2
  content and goals, 87–88
  lecture handout, 118–123
 session 3
  content and goals, 89–90
  lecture handout, 124–129
 session 4
  content and goals, 91–92
  lecture handout, 130–134
 session 5
  content and goals, 93
  lecture handout, 135–137
 session 6
  content and goals, 94–95
  lecture handout, 138–141
 session 7
  content and goals, 96–97
  lecture handout, 142–146

session 8
  content and goals, 98
  lecture handout, 147–151
session 9
  content and goals, 99–100
  lecture handout, 152–154
session 10
  content and goals, 101
  lecture handout, 155–159
session 11
  content and goals, 102–103
  lecture handout, 160–167
session 12
  content and goals, 104
  lecture handout, 168–171
session 13
  content and goals, 105
  lecture handout, 172–175
session 14
  content and goals, 106–107
  lecture handout, 176–184
session 15
  content and goals, 108
  lecture handout, 185–188
stress management, 102–103, 160–167
structure, 76–77
therapist qualifications, 76
therapist role, 77
treatment goals, 59–60, 75–76
weight loss treatment, 32–33
weight management, 105, 172–175
Cognitive functioning
  clinical conceptualization of BED, 8
  network of responses, 78, 130–131
  obesity as psychopathology, 24
  restructuring thoughts, 135–137
  styles of thinking, 132
  See also Cognitive-behavioral therapy
Cognitive restructuring, 62–63
Comorbidity in BED
  BED onset patterns and, 15
  medical complications, 39–41
  obesity and, 18, 27
  personality disorders, 22
  pharmacotherapy, 42
  psychopathology, 20–21
  research needs, 71
  risk, 18, 21
  therapeutic significance, 21
  treatment-seeking behavior and, 21
Comorbidity in obesity, 24
Consequences of behavior, 79–80, 118, 119, 120–121,
    138–141

Construct validity, 6
Content validity, 6
Control, loss of
  clinical conceptualization of BED, 3–4, 70
  cognitive-behavioral therapy, 96–97, 142–146
  etiological models of BED, 30, 70
  obesity as psychopathology, 24
  strategies for self-control, 142–143
Cortisol, 29
Course of BED, 16–17, 22
  onset, 13–15
  spontaneous remission, 16, 17
  weight gain, 16
  weight loss treatment and, 15
Cues and behavioral chains
  Cognitive-behavioral therapy, 14, 76, 77–78, 87–90,
      94–95, 118–119, 138–141
  external cues, 78
  internal cues, 78
  therapeutic goals, 79

Decision-analysis, 62
Depression
  associated medical problems, 40, 41
  binge eating to regulate, 15
  prevalence in BED, 18, 21
Desipramine, 42, 68
Fenfluramine, 44
Diabetes mellitus, 40–41, 48
Diagnosis
  alternative classifications for BED, 7–9
  BED diagnostic criteria, 3–7, 12, 35
  BED in children and adolescents, 11
  BED subtypes, 8
  dietary restraint, 17
  differential, 6–7
  obesity as psychopathology, 23–24
  subthreshold eating disorders, 6
Diagnostic and Statistical Manual of Mental Disorders,
    3, 4–5, 23, 70
Dialectal behavior therapy, 64, 65
Dieting behavior
  assessment, 13
  clinical features of BED, 17
  in early-onset BED, 11
  etiological model of BED, 27–28, 30, 124
  onset of BED, 13–15
  restraint/dieting model of BED, 13–15
  weight cycling, 29
  weight loss outcomes, 65
  See also Fasting; Weight loss treatment
Differential diagnosis, 6–7
Dimensional models of eating disorders, 7–8

Disability, obesity as psychopathology, 24
Distress
  assessment, 6
  BED diagnostic criteria, 6
  obesity as psychopathology, 24

Eating behavior
  diagnosing BED in children and adolescents, 11
  food deprivation effects, 36–37
  food presentation effects, 37
  patient self-monitoring, 80–81
  rate of eating, 36
  research challenges, 36
  research methods, 36, 37
  treatment goals, 124
  See also Binge-eating behavior; Patterns of
    overeating
Eating Behaviors Self-Monitoring Worksheet, 80–81,
    86, 88, 94, 114, 115
Eating Disorder Examination, 4
Eating disorder not otherwise specified, 16, 70
Ecological momentary assessment, 37–38, 67
Environmental factors in obesity, 31
  cues, 78
Epidemiology, 9–10, 12
  comorbidity in BED, 18, 21
  obesity and BED, 9, 25
Etiology
  BED subtypes based on onset patterns, 15
  body perception, 15, 148
  dieting behavior in origins of BED, 27–28, 30,
    124
  emotional regulation, 15
  multifactorial model, 58–59
  relationship between obesity and binge eating, 27–
    31
  restraint model, 13
  significance of obesity in BED, 23
Evolutionary theory, 124
Exercise, 67, 128
  Cognitive-behavioral therapy, 125–126, 172
Experiential learning, 63
Exposure-based intervention with body image, 67
Exposures for High Risk Foods Worksheet, 181–182
Exposures for High Risk Situations Worksheet, 183–
    184
Exposure to high risk foods and situations, 175, 176–
    177, 181–184

Fasting, 7, 124
  food deprivation effects on eating behavior, 36–37
  See also Dieting behavior
Fitness instruction, 67
Fluoxetine, 42–44, 46, 68

Fluvoxamine, 44, 68
Forbidden foods, 124

Gastric surgery. See Bariatric surgery
Gastroplasty, 50
Gender differences
  BED epidemiology, 10
  medical complications of BED, 39
Genetics
  BED risk, 38
  common risk factors for obesity and binge eating,
    30–31
  research needs, 71
Ghrelin, 29, 38
Grazing, 4, 55
Group therapy, weight loss treatment, 32–33
Guilt, 124

Health care utilization, 40
Healthy Exercise Worksheet, 89, 128
Healthy Lifestyle Plan, 188
Heart disease, 41
Hedonics of binge eating, 18
High Risk Foods and Situations Worksheet, 175
Hypertension, 40

Identifying Behavioral Chains Worksheet, 141
Imipramine, 42, 68
Impact of Weight on Quality of Life, 39–40
Incidence, BED, 9
International Classification of Diseases, 3
Interpersonal therapy, 63–64, 67
  effectiveness, 65

Jejunoileal bypass, 50

Lapse Plan and Relapse Plan Worksheet, 180
Learning to Handle Mistakes, 103, 165
Loss of loved one, BED onset patterns and, 15

Meal Plan Worksheet, 89–90, 129
Meditation, 64
Melanocortin-4 receptor, 30–31, 39
Mindfulness meditation, 64
Mood enhancement techniques, 143–144
Motivational enhancement therapy, 67
Musculoskeletal pain, 40

Negative self-evaluation as BED risk factor, 7
Nibbling, 4, 55
Nonbinge meals
  in BED, 13
  in BN, 13
Nonverbal communication, 169

Obesity and BED, 58–59
  associated psychopathology, 18
  calorie consumption in binge eating, 36
  in children and adolescents, 10–11
  clinical conceptualization of BED, 3, 8–9, 25–27, 70
  clinical significance, 17–18, 22, 23, 25–26, 31–33
  comorbid psychopathology and, 18, 20, 21
  direction of relationship, 27–31
  natural course, 16
  onset of BED, 15
  prevalence, 9, 25
  research needs, 33–34, 70, 71
  vulnerability to obesity as BED risk factor, 7
  See also Bariatric surgery
Obesity as eating disorder, 23–24
Objective episodes of binge eating, 4, 5
Obsessive–compulsive disorder, BED comorbidity, 22
Onset of BED, 13–15, 17
  etiological subtypes based on, 15
  therapeutic significance, 15
Orlistat, 45, 46, 68
Overeating. *See* Patterns of overeating

Pain, musculoskeletal, 40
Panic disorder, BED comorbidity, 21
Patterns of overeating
  in BED, 13, 59–60
  diagnostic criteria for BED, 4, 5, 6
  at nonbinge meals, 13
  obesity as psychopathology, 24
  onset of BED, 13–15
  weight cycling, 29
  See also Binge-eating behavior
Personality disorders
  BED comorbidity, 22
  See also specific disorder
Pharmacotherapy
  antidepressant therapy, 42–44, 48
  with psychotherapy, 46, 68, 69
  rationale, 41–42, 48
  treatment approach, 45–46
  weight loss agents, 44–45
Physiology. *See* Psychobiology
Picking, 4
Pleasant Activities Worksheet, 146
Positive energy balance, 29
Prevalence
  BED, 9–10
  comorbidity in BED, 18, 21
  obesity, 49
  obesity and BED, 9, 25
Preventive intervention
  BED relapse, 63, 76, 106–108, 176–188
  to prevent obesity, 15, 26, 33

Principles of Acceptance and Self-Acceptance, 103, 166
Psychobiology
  BED, 38–39
  cues, 78
  eating behavior leading to obesity, 29
  medical complications of BED, 39–41, 48
  obesity-related complications, 49
  research needs, 71
Psychodynamic interpersonal therapy, 65
Psychopathology, obesity as, 23–24
Purging
  in bulimia nervosa, 6
  nonpurging bulimia nervosa versus BED, 6–7

Quality of life
  bariatric surgery and, 52–53
  medical complications of BED, 39–40

Race/ethnicity
  BED epidemiology, 9–10
  body image concerns, 10
Rearranging Consequences: Goal-Setting and Self-Rewards Worksheet, 87, 88, 121, 123
Rearranging Cues Worksheet, 87–88, 89, 121, 122, 127
Reasons for and against Changing Unhealthy Eating Habits Worksheet, 85, 86, 114, 116
Relapse prevention, 63, 76, 106–108, 176–188
Relapse Scenario Worksheet, 179
Research needs
  BED in special populations, 12
  binge-eating behavior in BED, 70–71
  comorbidity, 71
  cultural factors, 71
  diagnosing BED in children and adolescents, 12
  obesity and BED, 33–34, 70, 71
  psychobiology of BED, 71
  psychosocial risk factors, 12
  treatment, 68–69
Response network, 77, 78–79, 130–131
Restraint theory, 13–15
Restructuring Thoughts Worksheet, 80–81, 92, 93, 134
Rewards, in cognitive-behavioral therapy, 120–121
Risk factors
  common factors for obesity and binge eating, 30–31
  exposure to high risk foods and situations, 175, 176–177, 181–184
  genetic, 30–31, 38–39
  obesity-related, 30
  psychosocial, 7, 12
  research needs, 70
Roux-en-Y gastric bypass, 50–51

Selective serotonin reuptake inhibitors, 42–44, 68
Self-Concept Inventory, 101, 156–157, 158–159

Self-esteem, 101, 155–159
Self-monitoring, in cognitive-behavioral therapy, 61, 80–81
Self-reports
    BED prevalence estimates based on, 9
    reliability of eating behavior reports, 5, 36
Self-talk, to develop assertiveness, 168–170
Serotonergic system, 38
Sertraline, 44
Sexual abuse
    BED onset patterns and, 15
    as BED risk factor, 7
Shyness as BED risk factor, 7
Sibutramine, 44–45
Sociocultural values
    body perception, 147–148, 150
    research needs, 71
    therapeutic considerations, 62–63
Statistical modeling of eating disorders, 7–8
Stress Reduction Experiment Worksheet, 103, 167
Stress response
    Cognitive-behavioral therapy, 102–103, 160–167
    physiology of weight gain, 29
Structured Interview for Anorexic and Bulimic Disorders, 4–5
Subjective episodes of binge eating, 4, 5
Subjective obesity, 58
Substance use disorder
    BED comorbidity and, 21
    BED onset patterns and, 15
Subthreshold eating disorders, 6

Taxometric analyses, 8
Thoughts Associated with Assertive and Nonassertive Behavior Worksheet, 104, 171
Three-Factor Eating Questionnaire, 13
Topiramate, 45

Treatment of BED
    age at onset and, 15
    augmentation strategies, 67–68
    combined medication and psychotherapy, 46, 68, 69
    comorbid psychopathology and, 21
    course of concurrent medical illness and, 41
    dialectal behavior therapy, 64
    implications of obesity, 25–26
    interpersonal therapy, 63–64, 65, 67
    mechanism of change, 58
    outcomes, 16, 17, 65–68, 75
    psychotherapeutic approaches, 58, 59
    research needs, 68–69, 71
    severity of BED and, 65
    treatment matching, 64–65
    See also Cognitive-behavioral therapy; Pharmacotherapy
Treatment of obesity
    implications of BED, 31–33
    See also Bariatric surgery; Weight loss treatment
Treatment-seeking behavior
    comorbidity in BED and, 21
    health care utilization, BED and, 40
    normal weight individuals with BED, 25
Tricyclic antidepressants, 42, 68

Validity of clinical model of BED, 6, 12
Very-low-calorie diets, 64
    adherence, 15

Weight loss treatment
    adherence, 15
    behavioral interventions, 64, 65, 67
    binge-eating behavior and, 15, 33
    clinical significance of BED, 32–33, 53
    cognitive-behavioral intervention, 105, 172–175
    outcomes research, 65
    pharmacotherapy, 44–45
    See also Bariatric surgery; Treatment of obesity